THERAPEUTIC REVOLUTION
The History of Medical Oncology from Early Days to the Creation of the Subspecialty

Authored By

Pierre R. Band

Department of Medicine
McGill University
Montreal
Canada

Art: From a painting by Alex Janvier, Native Canadian Artist. Author's collection

To the pioneers of medical oncology

To the patients who made it possible

Bentham Science Publishers
Executive Suite Y - 2
PO Box 7917, Saif Zone
Sharjah, U.A.E.
subscriptions@benthamscience.org

Bentham Science Publishers
P.O. Box 446
Oak Park, IL 60301-0446
USA
subscriptions@benthamscience.org

Bentham Science Publishers
P.O. Box 294
1400 AG Bussum
THE NETHERLANDS
subscriptions@benthamscience.org

CONTENTS

About the Author

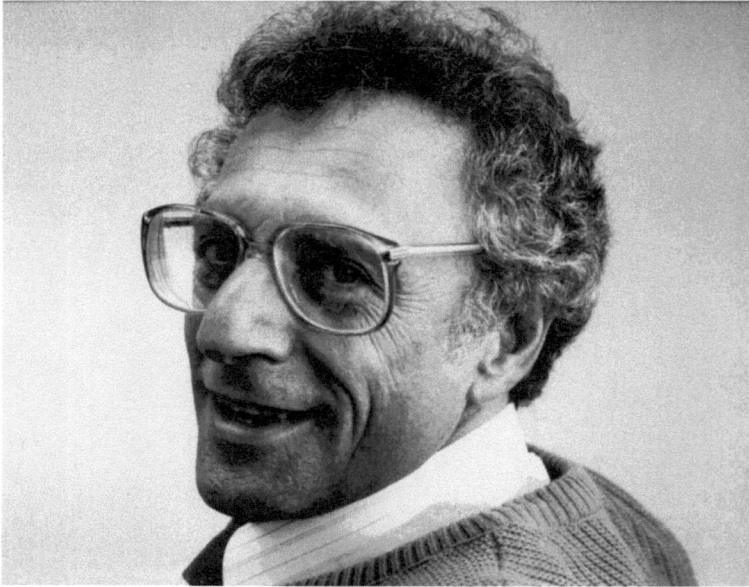

The author graduated from the Université de Montréal. He trained in medical oncology before the subspecialty was created, with Dr. Georges Mathé at the Institut Gustave-Roussy in France and with Dr. James F. Holland at Roswell Park Memorial Institute in the United States. He was a member of several Cooperative Oncology Groups, both in Europe and North America. Dr. Band wrote the protocol for the joint National Surgical Adjuvant Breast Project-Eastern Cooperative Oncology Group breast cancer study of postoperative ("adjuvant") L-phenylalanine mustard (L-PAM) chemotherapy. He was the first to use tamoxifen in North America as part of a Phase II clinical trial he designed for the treatment of metastatic breast cancer, to which clinical investigators in Europe and the United States participated.

FOREWORD

History is written by the victors. Although the vanquished may offer explanations, excuses or speculative essays on what it would have been like had they won, such efforts rarely depict reality. Often a victory is described by someone who was remote from the battle, a historian distant in time, with no passion and scars from the conflict. Pierre Band is not that kind of historian. He was fully engaged in the extraordinary turbulence that permeated the early years of medical oncology.

Surgery for cancer had existed for many hundreds of years, although anesthesia only appeared in the 1840s. Ovariectomy was introduced for breast cancer in the 1890s and castration for prostate cancer in the 1940s. Radiotherapy for cancer began in the early 1900s. Nitrogen mustards were explored as cancer drugs in the 1940s, under cover of wartime secrecy. The excitement really began in the late 1940s, when aminopterin was shown to induce temporary remissions in children with acute leukemia. Acute leukemia of children then became the first target of opportunity for scientists and doctors who were not surgeons. Principles of cancer chemotherapy were unraveled and chemotherapy began to be used in solid tumors immediately post-surgery and then before surgery, within the setting of rigorous clinical trials.

Dr. Band unfolds this fascinating story with the familiarly of a participant, drawing upon his correspondence and interviews with most of the main characters, and imbued with the excitement of this dynamic and revolutionary tale. The story of how a new discipline in medicine came about, bringing the promise of eventual triumph over cancer is among the great tales of the twentieth century.

This book tells that story. It is a record of struggle and triumph that sets the record straight. May it inspire young minds to pursue new quests to finish the task and open new vistas for improving the human condition.

James F. Holland, MD
Distinguished Professor of Neoplastic Diseases
The Derald H Ruttenberg Cancer Center
Mount Sinai School of Medicine
New York

PREFACE

Many books have been written about cancer and many articles have been published on the history of chemotherapy, but none to our knowledge on the history of medical oncology, that is, the events that led to this new subspecialty of internal medicine, which was first established in the United States in 1972. As a medical oncologist, I had been thinking of writing a book on this subject and discussed the idea with Dr. Roberto Zanetti, Director of the Piedmont Cancer Registry in Torino, Italy, with whom I had spent a mini-sabbatical. He encouraged me to go ahead, despite my hesitations as I am not a historian. Before deciding to proceed, however, I first wanted to test the ground by preparing a set of slides for potential lectures. Zanetti kindly invited me, with the financial contribution of the Fondo Anglesio Moroni in Torino, to give a series of talks in Torino, Parma and Florence, Italy. All my talks were well received.

Serendipity being what it is, I had read a paper by Dr. Franco Muggia discussing the screening of cancer chemotherapeutic agents, an important topic in the early days of medical oncology. Muggia and I were members of the Eastern Cooperative Oncology Group; although we had no contact for many years I phoned his office in October 2009, to tell him of my plans. Muggia, the Chairman of the annual Chemotherapy Foundation Symposium, invited me to speak at its XXVIIth conference, to be held the following month in New York City, a talk that was subsequently published [1]. There were about 2000 people in the audience, mostly medical oncologists and oncology nurses of various ages. I then gave a similar presentation in Montreal on receiving the "Pioneers in Canadian Oncology Award" from the Canadian Medical Oncology Association. Judging from the comments received, I realized that the history of medical oncology was a subject of great interest and possibly a gap to be filled, at least from the perspective of the younger generation.

Since my talks included an overview of the history of cancer that preceded the first modern treatment of malignant diseases, I intended to gain access to the Osler Library of the History of Medicine at McGill University in Montreal. To do so conveniently, for instance to access electronic material at the McGill libraries from home, I needed a Faculty appointment at McGill University. For this, I owe sincere thanks to Dr. Phil Gold, Professor of Physiology and Oncology at McGill University, who kindly arranged for me to be granted an appointment in the Department of Medicine.

At the same time, I had the chance to interview or talk on the phone to the pioneers who laid the foundations of medical oncology. A large part of this book relates their recollection of key events.

Pierre R. Band

Department of Medicine
McGill University
Montreal
Canada
E-mail: pierre.band@gmail.com

REFERENCE

[1]   Band PR. The birth of the subspecialty of medical oncology and examples of its early scientific foundations. J Clin Oncol 2010; 28:3653-8.

ACKNOWLEDGEMENTS

I cannot overemphasize my gratitude to everyone I have had the chance to contact or work with. Without them this book would not have been possible. They are: Doctors Gianni Bonadonna, Robert W. Bruce, Nicholas Bruchovsky, George Canellos, Paul P. Carbone, Bayard Clarkson, Andrew Coldman, Richard Cooper, Vincent De Vita, Bernard Fisher, Emil Frei III, Emil J. Freireich, Phil Gold, James Goldie, Thomas C. Hall, Jules Harris, James F. Holland, Jimmie C. Holland, John Kelsey, Lucien Israël, Irving Johnson, Irwin Krakoff, Harvey Lerner, Larry Norton, Georges Mathé, Franco Muggia, Hyman Muss, Albert Owens Jr., Joseph Ragaz, Maurice Schneider, Janet Wolter and Roberto Zanetti, as well as Lois Trench and Scott Kennedy.

Special thanks go to the McGill librarians for their ongoing assistance, and to John Stewart and Dr. Cornelia Hentzsch of Purdue Pharma, for a grant that enabled me to meet, interview and film Doctors Frei, Freireich and Holland. I am indebted to Diana Thiriar and to Christian Band for grammatical and other editing and to Helmut Bernhard of Neuro Media Services at McGill University for his professional help with the iconographic material and also for contributing his expert touch to improve the photographs that I took.

I owe particular gratitude to my mentor Dr. James F. Holland for his editorial comments and numerous helpful suggestions, to my friend and colleague Dr. Nicholas Bruchovsky for his painstaking editing of the entire book and to Kathe Lieber for professional editing of the final text.

There is no conflict of interest for the ebook.

CHAPTER 1

The Author Introduces Himself

Pierre R. Band[*]

Department of Medicine, McGill University, Montreal, Canada

Abstract: During his internship in 1961, the author sent letters of inquiry asking which centers in the United States provided a residency program in cancer medicine and what kind of training was offered. The answers were unexpected. Not only did these simple questions appear to be difficult to answer, but one reply indicated that a cancer specialist was a non-entity! The author briefly describes the training he received from two of his mentors, Dr. Georges Mathé in France, and Dr. James F. Holland in the United States, exemplifying what existed at the time when the methodology of clinical trials was being developed and the experimental bases of chemotherapy were being conceived and tested within the setting of cooperative oncology groups.

Keywords: Training in cancer medicine, clinical trials, experimental chemotherapy.

INTRODUCTION

I was born in Paris to Hungarian parents and immigrated to Canada when I was 15, leaving behind close friends at an age when identification with a group takes on major importance. The shock must have been violent: I became a high-school dropout and worked at a restaurant in Montreal called Bens that was famous for its smoked meat sandwiches. After a year of preparing smoked meat and pickles I decided to go back to school, working very hard to compensate for the time lost. It took courage from the professor who interviewed me to allow me to enter medical school at the Université de Montréal, considering my unorthodox track record. During my internship in 1961, I pondered what career to pursue. I did not want to follow common paths nor specialize in diseases of a single organ, such as the heart, or a system, such as the gastrointestinal tract, but wished to remain close to internal medicine. And so I opted for cancer medicine. It was an easy decision: there was little else to choose from and it did not exist! One of the professors of pathology, who was on the Board of the National Cancer Institute of Canada, advised me to apply for a fellowship and suggested that I should consider the Institut Gustave-Roussy, the main cancer center in France.

*Address correspondence to Pierre R. Band: Faculty of Medicine, McGill University, Montreal, Quebec H3G 1Y6, Canada; E-mail: pierre.band@gmail.com

I also sent out letters of inquiry asking two simple questions: what centers in the United States provided a residency in cancer medicine and what kind of training program they offered. The replies were unexpected. The American Medical Association informed me that "There are no longer any formal residency training programs in cancer, malignant diseases or oncology" (Fig. **1.1**). If that first answer was not very encouraging, I was bewildered by the second, from the American

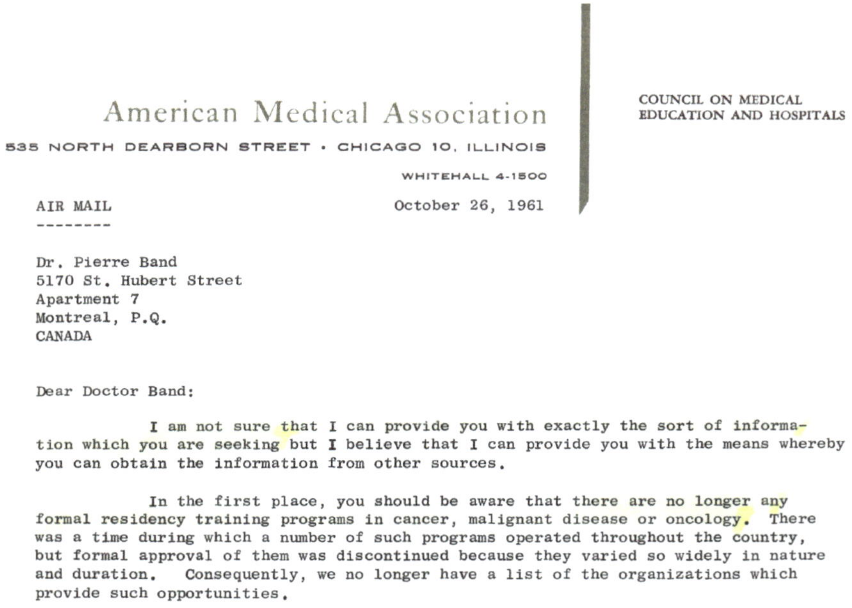

American Medical Association
535 NORTH DEARBORN STREET • CHICAGO 10, ILLINOIS
WHITEHALL 4-1500

COUNCIL ON MEDICAL EDUCATION AND HOSPITALS

AIR MAIL

October 26, 1961

Dr. Pierre Band
5170 St. Hubert Street
Apartment 7
Montreal, P.Q.
CANADA

Dear Doctor Band:

I am not sure that I can provide you with exactly the sort of information which you are seeking but I believe that I can provide you with the means whereby you can obtain the information from other sources.

In the first place, you should be aware that there are no longer any formal residency training programs in cancer, malignant disease or oncology. There was a time during which a number of such programs operated throughout the country, but formal approval of them was discontinued because they varied so widely in nature and duration. Consequently, we no longer have a list of the organizations which provide such opportunities.

Figure 1.1: Letter received from the American Medical Association.

Cancer Society: "First off, there really isn't any recommended special training for oncology because the clinical and oncologic specialty system of medical practice determines the course of treatment of the cancer patient, thus making a 'cancer specialist' a non-entity" (Fig. **1.2**). Finally, what I thought were straightforward questions seemed difficult to answer, judging from the reply I received from the National Institutes of Health (Fig. **1.3**). Despite this discouraging news, I went on to spend several years of training in cancer medicine in the departments of Dr. Georges Mathé (Fig. **1.4**) at the Institut Gustave-Roussy, Villejuif, France, and Dr. James F. Holland (Fig. **1.5**) at Roswell Park Memorial Institute, Buffalo, New York. I owe to

American Cancer Society, Inc. / **Research · Education · Service**

521 West 57 Street, New York 19, New York PLaza 7-2700

November 20, 1961

Dr. Pierre Band
5170 St. Hubert Street
Apartment 7
Montreal, P.Q.

Dear Dr. Band:

I have your letter of November 12, 1961 requesting
information concerning your training in "clinical
oncology." As you indicated your questions are
quite broad and my answers will have to be the same.

First off, there really isn't any recommended special
training for oncology because the clinical and oncologic specialty system of medical practice determines
the course of treatment of the cancer patient, thus
making a "cancer specialist" a non-entity. One can
become a so-called clinical cancerologist only inso-
far as he is an internist or a surgeon, clinical
pathologist, radiologist, etc. I would assume from
your letter that you are primarily interested in
internal medicine, and therefore your proposed course
of internal medicine, one year of pathology is a
good one. I would strongly suggest that you could
best decide what sort of training you needed if you
had an opportunity to visit several outstanding cancer
institutions. It would be a good idea to plan to
visit the Roswell Park Memorial Institute in Buffalo,
New York. Dr. George Moore is the Director and I'm
sure that he would be pleased to have you visit the
Institution and discuss with you the matter of your
training.

Similarly, a trip to Memorial Cancer Center in New
York City would be recommended. While in New York
you could also visit the Delafied Hospital of
Columbia Presbyterian Medical Center. Anyone of
these three institutions could provide you with
excellent training for the type of future you envision.

Sincerely,

Roald N. Grant, M. D.
Director of Professional
Education

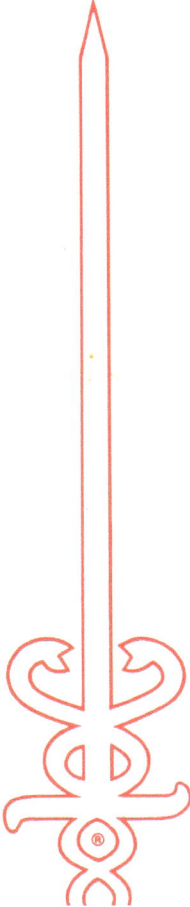

Figure 1.2: Letter received from the American Cancer Society.

these mentors the opportunity to have lived, and contributed to some of the most exciting and stimulating pioneering years of medical oncology. Those were the days when the methodology of clinical trials was being developed and the experimental bases of chemotherapy were being conceived and tested within the setting of cooperative oncology groups. The torch of knowledge is passed from one generation to the next. Holland and Mathé belonged to the first generation of pioneers in oncology. I had the good fortune of being among the second, close to the precursors, many of whom I had the chance to meet.

In turn, I would like to share with the younger generation of medical oncologists a personal overview of what paved the way for the specialty they have elected to embrace.

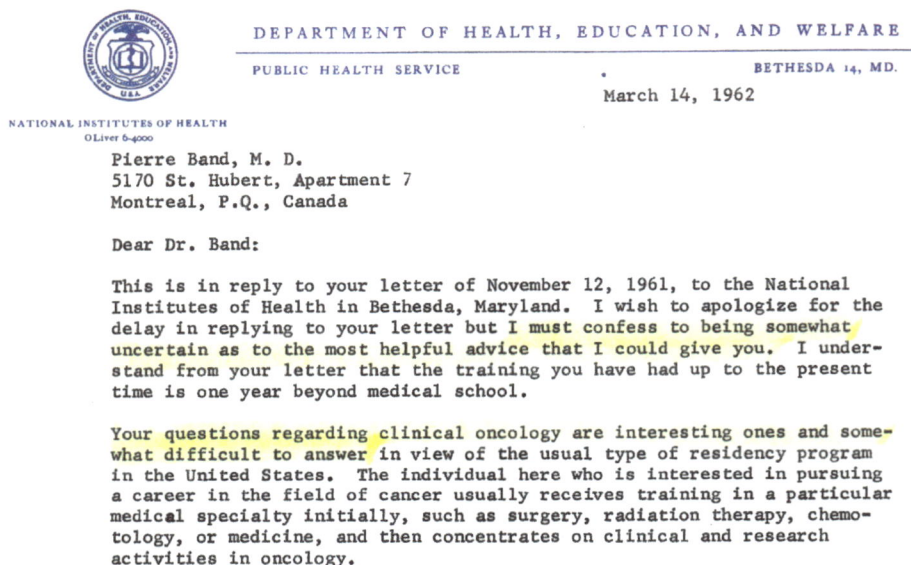

DEPARTMENT OF HEALTH, EDUCATION, AND WELFARE

PUBLIC HEALTH SERVICE   BETHESDA 14, MD.

March 14, 1962

NATIONAL INSTITUTES OF HEALTH
OLiver 6-4000

Pierre Band, M. D.
5170 St. Hubert, Apartment 7
Montreal, P.Q., Canada

Dear Dr. Band:

This is in reply to your letter of November 12, 1961, to the National Institutes of Health in Bethesda, Maryland. I wish to apologize for the delay in replying to your letter but I must confess to being somewhat uncertain as to the most helpful advice that I could give you. I understand from your letter that the training you have had up to the present time is one year beyond medical school.

Your questions regarding clinical oncology are interesting ones and somewhat difficult to answer in view of the usual type of residency program in the United States. The individual here who is interested in pursuing a career in the field of cancer usually receives training in a particular medical specialty initially, such as surgery, radiation therapy, chemotology, or medicine, and then concentrates on clinical and research activities in oncology.

Figure 1.3: Letter received from the National Institutes of Health.

Mathé, who died in 2010 at the age of 88, was a hematologist and immunologist who took postgraduate training in immunology and oncology at Memorial Sloan-Kettering Cancer Center in New York City. He became recognized worldwide not only for having performed the first bone marrow transplant in non-identical twins, but for the very unusual circumstances under which the procedure was initially accomplished: the treatment of Yugoslavian physicists who had been irradiated during a nuclear reactor accident [1]. In 1961, Mathé became head of the Department of Hematology at the Institut Gustave-Roussy, where he carried out experimental and clinical research in bone marrow transplant for the treatment of acute leukemia and other malignancies. Mathé was one of the founding members and first president of the *Groupe européen de chimiothérapie anticancéreuse,* a clinical cooperative oncology group that became the European Organization for Research and Treatment of Cancer (EORTC) in 1965. With Dr. Maurice

Schneider, one of his former staffmen, he founded the European Society for Medical Oncology in the mid-seventies.

I arrived in Mathé's department in July 1964 after two years of residency in internal medicine in Montreal. As a resident (or intern, as they are called in France), I was responsible for about 25 inpatients, mostly children and adults with acute leukemia. I had the opportunity to learn about this disease, its dreadful complications and the familial impact of malignancies, and to participate in clinical trials of investigational chemotherapeutic agents, some of which were part of the *Groupe européen de chimiothérapie anticancéreuse* studies.

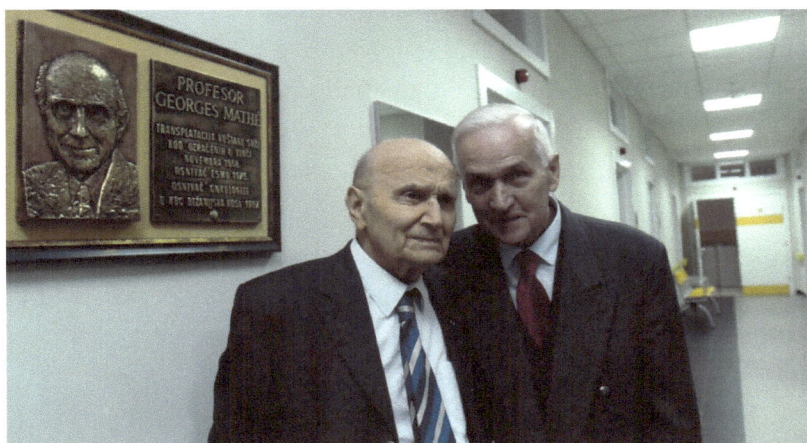

Figure 1.4: Dr. Georges Mathé (left) and Maksic Radojko, one of the Yugoslavian nuclear physicists who underwent the first bone marrow transplantation in January 1958. Photo taken at the inauguration of the Georges Mathé Cancer Center in Belgrade in 2007. Photo taken and kindly provided to the author by Michelle Chaker, Executive Secretary, Institut André Lwoff, Villejuif, France.

In January 1966, I joined the department of Dr. James F. Holland, Chief, Medicine A, at Roswell Park Memorial Institute, as a National Institutes of Health Post-Graduate Fellow. Holland's contributions to cancer medicine will figure prominently in this book. Suffice it to say here that Holland was the first attending physician at the National Cancer Institute when the National Institutes of Health in Bethesda, Maryland, opened its Clinical Center, where he developed what was to become the first-ever clinical cooperative trial in childhood acute leukemia. Holland was a founding member of the Acute Leukemia Group B (ALGB), which he chaired from 1963 to 1981.

Adjacent to his small office was a slightly bigger room, essentially occupied by a table where the staff, fellows and residents used to crowd together when he wanted to share important information with them. It was there that one day I asked Holland what my project would be. He pulled from the pocket of his white coat a small plastic container filled with pills, placed it in the middle of the table, told me this was my project and left. The container had a number written on it: NSC 29630; so I went to the pharmacy department to ask whether the number was by any chance linked to other less cryptic information. After being told that the pills were called dichloromethotrexate, I informed Holland of what he already knew. He told me I should carry out a Phase II study of that compound. Since I had little knowledge of how to do that, I read up intensively on the methodology of experimental and clinical drug evaluation and whatever was known of NSC 29630. When Holland and I met again in that same room, he must have been pleased with my progress, because he told me to write a Phase II protocol for the drug in question, carry out the study in lung-cancer patients and write a paper. Before leaving, as a token of his appreciation, Holland wrote the following words on a slip of paper: introduction, method, results, discussion, conclusion. The study was done and published. This is a true account of what happened, and I regret to say that this type of training has largely been forgotten.

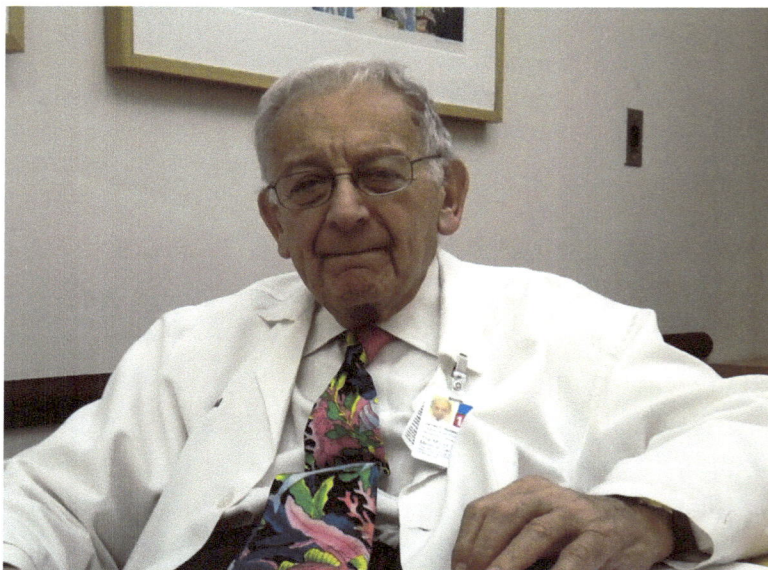

Figure 1.5: Dr. James F. Holland. Photo taken by the author; New York City, November 2010.

In 1968, before returning to Canada, I applied for positions in medical oncology. Once again, the replies were unexpected. The head of the Department of Medicine at a major teaching hospital where one hematologist was treating cancer patients told me that "two cancer specialists would step on each others' toes". The most laudatory reply came from a provincial Canadian Cancer Center stating that I was overqualified for the job. Cancer medicine must not have been considered to be a very attractive profession. This was the situation at the time in Canada, while in the United States comprehensive cancer centers and separate divisions of oncology were being set up, offering career opportunities to many young oncologists, including several of my Canadian colleagues.

At last a positive answer arrived from the University of Alberta in Edmonton, which I joined in July 1969. My first undertaking was to apply for membership in the Eastern Cooperative Oncology Group (ECOG); the University of Alberta thus became the first Canadian center affiliated with this group. I also became a member of the EORTC. While in Edmonton, I became involved in therapeutic trials in breast cancer that will be discussed in later chapters of this book. An important development at the time was the discovery of the carcinoembryonic antigen by Doctors Samuel Freedman and Phil Gold at McGill University in Montreal. It was hoped that a test of this antigen in the blood would make it possible to diagnose colon cancer at an early stage. I participated in collaborative studies investigating this antigen and heard a presentation by a cytopathologist, Dr. Geno Saccomanno (1915-1999), stating that there was a positive association between titers of the carcinoembryonic antigen and the degree of sputum cytology abnormalities. Saccomanno (Fig. **1.6**) began his career on the Colorado Plateau, where a number of uranium mines were operating. By taking serial sputum cytology samples from underground miners, he had described the development of lung cancer from normal cells to mild, moderate and severe atypias, to cancer *in situ* and invasive cancer [2], receiving the Papanicolaou Award for his work.

Since there was a uranium mine in the north of the province of Saskatchewan, with a company plane flying daily from Edmonton to the mine, I approached Saccomanno, asking him if he would be interested in a joint study investigating the role of the carcinoembryonic antigen and sputum cytology for the early detection of lung cancer in this high risk group. He agreed, and we conducted a study [3, 4] that would have a considerable influence on my career. First, because several cases of moderate and marked atypias where found among the miners we studied, I became interested in chemoprevention and the potential cancer-preventive effect of vitamin A and its synthetic analogs, which had been the subject of a recent publication [5]. Second, contacts with uranium workers gave me a keen interest in occupational health issues.

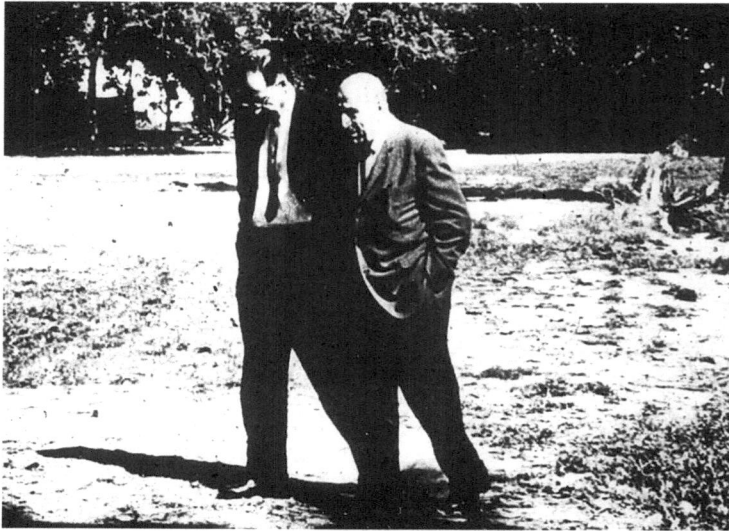

Figure 1.6: Doctors Geno Saccomanno (left) and George Papanicolaou, the father of cytology. Photo taken in February 1962, when Dr. Saccomanno received the Papanicolaou Award, 9 days before Dr. Papanicolaou's death. Photo kindly given to the author by Dr. Saccomanno.

This brought me to the British Columbia Cancer Agency in Vancouver in 1982 to set up a program in occupational cancer epidemiology, which became my main activity, although I continued to work as a medical oncologist, but in a more limited manner. I was surrounded by outstanding colleagues and friends among them Doctors Nicholas Bruchovsky and James Goldie (Fig. **1.7**).

Bruchovsky's demonstration that dihydrotestosterone is the active form of testosterone in the prostate radically changed notions of androgen physiology and physiopathology [6, 7]. Goldie's mathematical model developed with the statistician Dr. Andrew Coldman, triggered worldwide interest in the preoperative chemo-therapy or neoadjuvant approach to cancer treatment [8].

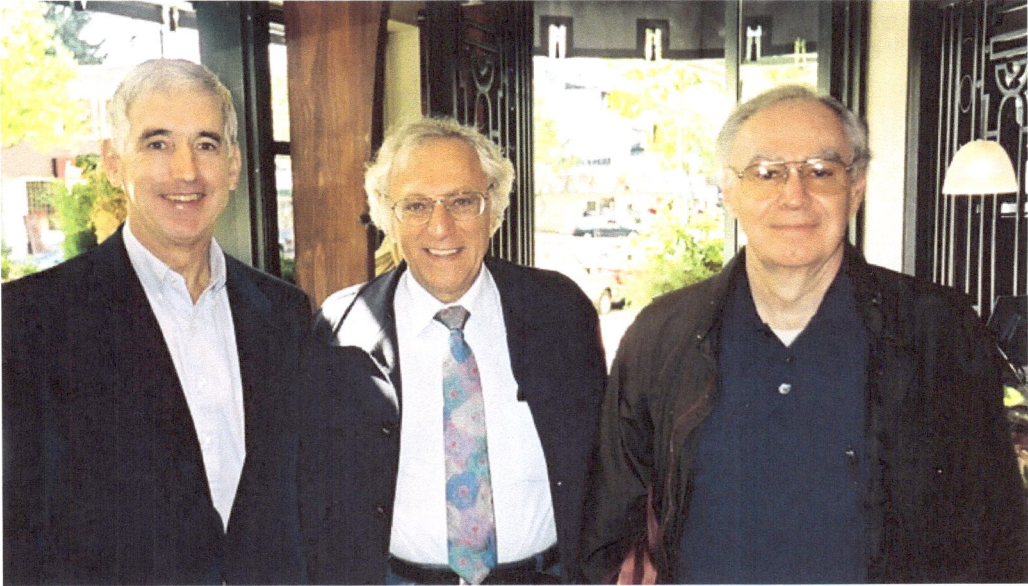

Figure 1.7: From left to right: Doctors Nicholas Bruchovsky, Pierre Band and James Goldie; Vancouver, 1998. Author's collection.

I left the Agency in 1996. The years spent there count among the most memorable of my professional life.

REFERENCES

[1]   Mathé G, Jammet H, Pendic B, *et al*. Transfusions and grafts of homologous bone marrow in humans after accidental high dosage irradiation. Rev Fr Etud Clin Biol 1959; 4:226-38.

[2]   Saccomanno G. Diagnostic Pulmonary Cytology. Chicago: American Society of Clinical Pathologists, 1978.

[3]   Band P, Feldstein M, Saccomanno G, Watson L, King G. Potentiation of cigarette smoking and radiation: evidence from a sputum cytology survey among uranium miners and controls. Cancer 1980; 45:1273-7.

[4]   Band P, Watson L, Saccomanno G, *et al*. Sputum cytology and carcinoembryonic (CEA) survey of uranium workers. In: Herbert E. Nieburgs, Ed. Prevention and Detection of Cancer. New York, Marcel Dekker, Inc., 1978; pp. 671-82.

[5]   Sporn MB, Dunlop NM, Newton DL, Smith JM. Prevention of chemical carcinogenesis by vitamin A and its synthetic analogs (retinoids). Fed Proc 1976; 35:1332-8.

[6]   Bruchovsky N, Wilson JD. The conversion of testosterone to 5α-androstan-17β-ol-3-one by rat prostrate *in vivo* and *in vitro*. J Biol Chem 1968; 243:2012-21.

[7]   Bruchovsky N, Wilson JD. Discovery of the role of dihydrotestosterone in androgen action. Steroids 1999; 64:753-9.

[8]   Goldie JH, Coldman AJ. A mathematic model for relating the drug sensitivity of tumors to their spontaneous mutation rate. Cancer Treat Rep 1979; 63:1727-33.

"It is better not to treat patients with deep-seated cancers; if treated, they die rapidly;
if not treated, they live longer". Hippocrates.

CHAPTER 2

From Dinosaurs to the Dawn of Chemotherapy: A Brief Overview

Pierre R. Band[*]

Department of Medicine, McGill University, Montreal, Canada

Abstract: A brief overview is presented, from early findings of malignant tumors to the beginning of modern chemotherapy. The humoral, lymphatic and cell theories of cancer are summarized, as well as major scientific developments and discoveries in medicine and oncology, such as anatomy, physiology and pathology, inhalation anesthesia, radiation and hormonal procedures. The contributions made by key scientists and physicians are emphasized.

Keywords: Humoral theory, lymphatic theory, cell theory, anesthesia, radiation, hormonal procedures.

INTRODUCTION

Although the history of modern medical oncology dates back little over half a century, cancer diseases have long been present. Evidence for the antiquity of malignant tumors comes from fossilized bone material and mummies and from early written documents. Primary and metastatic bone tumors have been found, albeit extremely rarely, in fossilized bones of dinosaurs and other animals [1-5], and have been recognized in Ancient Egypt and in the Pre-Columbian Incas [6-8]. Autopsies, radiographies and biopsies of mummies and other bone remains have shown involvement with various cancers, most commonly nasopharyngeal and multiple myeloma, but also with other types [6-8]. The first written record of cancer comes from the Edwin Smith papyrus of Ancient Egypt, where a case of breast cancer was reported with a comment that there was no treatment [9].

*Address correspondence to Pierre R. Band: Faculty of Medicine, McGill University, Montreal, Quebec H3G 1Y6, Canada; E-mail: pierre.band@gmail.com

THE HUMORAL THEORY OF CANCER

Cancer medicine in its conceptual aspects may be traced to Ancient Greece, where medicine was practiced by physicians instead of priests, as was generally the custom in Mesopotamia and Ancient Egypt. Reason replaced faith and superstition, and diseases became attributable to natural causes rather than to the wrath of the Gods: "Each disease has a natural cause and without a natural cause none occur" [author's translation, reference 10]. The term "*onco*," which became the root of the word *oncology*, referred to swellings or masses of any origin, whether malignant or not. The Greek physician Hippocrates (460 BC-375 BC) coined the term *karkinos*, meaning crab, for malignant tumors; the name likely comes from malignant tumors' resemblance to the shape of a crab, with a hard round center and leg-like projections. Hippocrates described visible or readily palpable cancers including those of the skin, head and neck, breast and cervix. His descriptions of virilization in two women who died of their disease are of special interest: "Menstruation ceased and the body took on a virile appearance, this woman became hairy all over, she grew a beard, her voice acquired harshness . . . this woman died in a short time" [author's translation, reference 11]. These cases (the second woman had the same clinical findings) may be the first-ever reported of virilizing ovarian or adrenal cancers, which at that time could not be diagnosed as such.

The cause of cancer was based on the theory of humors. This theory originated from the School of Pythagoras, which considered the number four, the sum and product of two equal numbers, to represent nature's perfection. That number became associated with the four universal elements, air, earth, water and fire, to which were added four qualities, dry, moist, cold and hot. The Hippocratic School added the four body humors, blood, phlegm, yellow bile and black bile, to the four universal elements and their qualities.

These humors were assumed to constitute the nature of the human body. The body is in a healthy state when the four humors are in equilibrium; diseases occur when one is reduced or in excess, or when it metastasizes, that is when it separates from the other humors and becomes confined to some part of the body [12]. Cancer was thought to be caused by an excess or sequestration of black bile [13, 14]. A number of practices aimed at expelling the harmful humor from the body, such as purging, bleeding and using emetics, are based on the humoral theory. As a child, I can recall that leeches were sold in pharmacies and that my grandmother used to apply cupping glasses on my back whenever I had a cold. The four humors were also linked to psychological characteristics and we still use such words as sanguine, phlegmatic, bilious and melancholic (from *melan chole*: black bile).

We owe the Latin word *cancer* to another Greek physician, Aulus Cornelius Celsus (30 BC-circa 38 AD), who practiced in Rome after Greece became part of the Roman Empire. His eight-volume treatise *De Medicina*, written in Latin, is an in-depth account of the medical and surgical knowledge from the time of Hippocrates. In his books, Celsus refers to several primary cancers and mentions the progression of cancer from an early tumor to an ulcerated one: "And generally the first stage is what the Greeks call *cacoethes* (malignant); then from that follows a carcinoma without ulceration; then ulceration, and from that a kind of wart [15]". Celsus further commented that with the exception of the first stage, cancer is incurable, as recurrence occurs even after a scar has formed [15], adding that the distinction between potentially curable cancers from incurable cancers can only be learned with time and experience. *De Medicina* was published in Florence in 1478, becoming the first printed book of medicine [14].

The third Greek physician to achieve celebrity as an outstanding practitioner and writer was Claudius Galen (130 AD-200 AD). His medical and surgical knowledge and skills made him the appointed physician to the gladiators, and the physician of two Roman emperors. His short book *De Tumoribus Praeter Naturam*, On Tumors beyond Nature, is devoted to swellings with diverse causes, including cancer. Galen followed and emphasized Hippocrates' humoral theory of cancer [14]. He considered two types of black bile, a milder form causing non-ulcerated cancer and another leading to ulceration: "When black bile attacks flesh, being biting it eats the surrounding skin and causes an ulcer; but when it is milder it causes cancer without ulceration [16]". Note the wording: attacks, bites, eats; these and similar words have remained attached to this disease. Galen's influence on medicine was considerable and his authoritative writings became dogma, to a large extent impeding medical progress during the Middle Ages.

Cancer treatment in Antiquity consisted of excision and cauterization with a hot iron of tumors deemed operable. For ulcerated cancer, ointments containing arsenic and vinegar and caustic pastes made of lime, arsenic, or various metals, including lead, copper, zinc or their salts, as well as soothing substances such as zinc oxide, cabbage or carrots mixed with honey, oil or other compounds, were applied as plasters [3, 17-20]. To ease pain, ointments made of poppy heads were used [17]. A number of other remedies, often complex mixtures made of minerals and various extracts of herbs, plants, trees, and even extracts from animals, were taken as infusions or used as external or internal applications [18-20]. It is difficult to assess the effectiveness of these medications, but zinc oxide applied to irritated skin is an effective soothing and anti-inflammatory compound, as every mother familiar with diaper rash can testify, and arsenic was still considered an effective caustic agent in the 18th century [17]. Similarly, mustard was used in the 16th and 17th century as a caustic and vesicant to treat cancer [17]; when I was a child, mustard poultices were still applied on the thorax as a lung decongestant and if care was not exercised, produced skin burns and blisters. However, the physicians of the time must have considered these remedies as palliative only, since potentially curable cancers were treated by non-medical means.

After the fall of the Roman Empire and the Barbarian invasions, Greco-Roman culture faded in Western Europe. It was Islam that preserved the Greco-Roman heritage. Beginning in the 7th century, Islam conquered an empire extending from Persia to Spain. Muslim scholars translated into Arabic, among other works, the Hippocratic Collection and Galen's books [21-25], and medicine flourished. For example, Avicenna's (987-1037) *Canon of Medicine* became a reference for several centuries, and Arabic physicians contributed to several medical fields including pharmacology and anesthesia [26, 27]. Starting with the reconquest of Spain by Christians and the Crusades, the Greco-Roman roots of Arabic medicine made their way back to Latin Europe through translations into Latin of Arabic manuscripts, chiefly the work of Hippocrates and Galen, by scholars from Salerno, Italy, and the College of Translators in Toledo, Spain [21, 22].

THE FOUNDATON OF SCIENCIFIC MEDICINE: NEW THERAPEUTIC MODALITIES

Major scientific achievements took place from the beginning of the Renaissance. Treatises by Vesalius (1514-1564*), De Humani Corporis Fabrica*, published in

1543, and William Harvey (1578-1657), *De Motu Cordis* published in 1628, set the foundations for human anatomy and physiology respectively. The lymphatic system was described between 1622 and 1652 by Gasparo Aselli (1581-1626), Jean Pecquet (1622-1674), Olaus Rudbeck (1630-1702) and Thomas Bartholin (1616-1680). That discovery led to the lymphatic theory of cancer proposed by René Descartes (1595-1650) and espoused by the French surgeon Henri-Francois Le Dran (1685-1770), whereby cancer was thought to be caused by fermented acidic lymph [13, 17, 28-30]. Not only did this theory put a dent in the theory of humors, but cancer came to be viewed as a local disease before spreading through the lymphatics; and so cancer could be cured if it was removed before the *levain cancéreux*, the cancerous yeast, infected the lymphatic system and entered the circulation [28]. This concept was destined to have far reaching consequences.

The Italian physician Giovanni Battista Morgagni (1682-1771), correlated clinical symptoms with autopsy findings. His book *De Sedibus et Causis Morborum per Anatomen Indagatis*, published in 1761, laid the groundwork for pathological anatomy, while the work of Marie-François-Xavier Bichat (1771-1802) on the composition of tissues established the basis of modern histology [29, 30]. The 19th century saw the emergence of cellular pathology, largely due to the German School. Johannes Müller (1801-1858) postulated that cancers were composed of cells [13, 29, 30], and his pupil Theodor Schwann (1810-1882), with Matthias Schleiden (1804-1881), developed the cell theory, whereby cells constitute the structural unit of life [30-32]. These authors, however, believed that cells arose spontaneously from an amorphous substance, which they called *blastema* [30, 32]. Rudolph Virchow (1821-1902) established that cells formed the basic biological unit in health and disease. His monumental achievements were the foundation of modern cellular pathology, forcefully summarized in his famous aphorism *omnis cellula e cellula*, meaning that all cells, including cancer cells, come from cells [17, 29, 31]. His work put an end to the humoral theory of cancer conceived 2000 years before.

These achievements were not paralleled by therapeutic advances in cancer treatment, with the exception of the considerable development of surgery that followed the introduction of inhalation anesthesia in 1846 and the use of antisepsis by Joseph Lister (1843-1910) in 1867, subsequent to the work of Louis Pasteur (1822-1898)

[33, 34]. The end of the 19th century, however, was marked by the discovery of X-rays in 1895 by Wilhelm Röntgen (1845-1923) [35], soon followed by the first use of X-rays for the treatment of breast cancer in 1896 [36]. That year also saw the introduction of bilateral ovariectomy for the treatment of advanced breast cancer, by George Thomas Beatson (1848-1933), a disciple of Lister [37]. This approach, which pioneered therapeutic endocrine procedures, represents the first form of effective systemic modality in the treatment of cancer. Beatson's remark that "one organ holding the control over the secretion of another separate organ . . . (in) the absence of distinct nervous control [37]" was a brilliant intuition of endocrine function. The reasons for performing this new surgical procedure in breast cancer were derived from Beatson's medical thesis on lactation. He observed that cell proliferation in the breast of lactating sheep was akin to cell proliferation in cancer "but in the case of lactation they rapidly vacuolate, undergo fatty degeneration and form milk; while in the carcinoma they stop short of that process, and, to make room for themselves, they penetrate the walls of the ducts and the acini and invade the surrounding tissues. In short, lactation is at one point perilously near becoming a cancerous process if it is at all arrested [37]". He also knew that removal of the ovaries from cows after calving prolonged milk production indefinitely. Hence the question: "Is cancer of the mamma due to some ovarian irritation . . . and, if so, would the cell proliferation be brought to a standstill, or would the cells go on to the fatty degeneration seen in lactation were the ovaries to be removed [37]?" It was with that hope that Beatson performed the first bilateral ovariectomy in a woman with a large chest wall recurrence and multiple skin nodules following radical mastectomy. The patient improved considerably. Also in 1896, Henry Becquerel (1852-1906) discovered the phenomenon of radioactivity, a term coined by Marie Curie (1867-1934) who, with her husband Pierre Curie (1859-1906), isolated radium in 1898; the application of radium was later used to treat cancer [38, 39]. Marie and Pierre Curie were awarded the Nobel Prize in Physics in 1903. Thus the end of the 19th century saw the birth of two new and effective forms of cancer treatment since the advent of surgery.

PAUL EHRLICH: AN INCOMPARABLE GENIUS

Paul Ehrlich (1854-1915) stands out as a unique creator who brought organic chemistry into biological science. He was an innovator in several branches of modern medicine, including hematology, immunology and infectious diseases. We owe to his studies of organic dyes, among others, the discovery of the mast cell, the differential staining of the neutrophil, basophil and eosinophil granulocytes, the classification of leukemias into myeloid and lymphoid, and the acid-fast staining of the tubercle bacillus. His work on the diphtheria antitoxin led him to develop the concept of a cell receptor to which the toxin becomes chemically linked, which he summarized in the aphorism *corpora non agunt nisi fixate*, substances don't act unless fixed. He considered the specific effect of toxins akin to a "magic bullet" searching and killing the invader. As few infectious diseases could be treated by immunological means, Ehrlich turned his attention to the treatment of infections with chemical agents, creating and naming a new field: chemotherapy. He investigated the effects of a number of dyes and arsenical compounds; among the former, trypan red cured the trypanosome responsible for diseases in horses, while the 606th compound of the latter, salvarsan, cured human syphilis.

In the course of these investigations, Ehrlich introduced the concept of "therapeutic index," the ratio of a toxic to a therapeutic dose, described the phenomenon of drug resistance and suggested combination chemotherapy as a means to circumvent it [40-42]. As Ehrlich elegantly stated: "Now, it is a frequent practice of many uncivilised people, in order to be certain of killing their enemies, that they not only rub over their arrow with one kind of poison, but with two or three totally different kinds of poison. And so it also appeared advisable to imitate this procedure against the parasites . . . and to poison our synthetically poisoned arrows not singly but doubly [43]" and: "combined therapy is best carried out with therapeutic agents which attack entirely different chemo-receptors in the parasites . . . but it is necessary to select from each group the most effective substance and then to combine the most suitable representatives of the various types. It is clear that in this manner a simultaneous and varied attack is directed on the parasites, in accordance with the military maxim: 'March apart but fight combined' [43]". Fifty years later, these pharmacologic principles would become part of cancer chemotherapy. Interestingly, it was Alphonse Laveran (1845-1922) who in 1902 first used this therapeutic approach against experimental trypanosomal infections in rodents; a combination of trypan red and arsenous acid cured the disease, whereas either compound alone failed to do so [44]. Laveran discovered the parasite that causes malaria and received the Nobel Prize in Physiology or Medicine in 1907, one year before Paul Ehrlich was given the Nobel for his work on immunology.

RADIATION THERAPY AND HORMONES

In the first half of the 20th century, the advances of the 19th century continued. Great progress was made in radiation therapy, especially with the advent of supervoltage radiation [36, 39]. New hormonal treatments were introduced for the treatment of prostate and breast cancer. Charles Huggins (1901-1997), a Canadian, pursued a brilliant career as a urologist and researcher at the University of Chicago Medical School, where he pioneered the use of antiandrogen treatment for prostate cancer. He showed that levels of acid phosphatases were stimulated by androgens and inhibited by estrogens and by bilateral orchiectomy [45].

Tumor regression and symptomatic benefit, particularly bone pain reduction, were noted following castration: "The improvement was greater than we have observed in any case in which far advanced or metastatic cancer was treated in any other way [46]". Based on the rationale that adrenal androgens may stimulate the growth of prostate cancer, Huggins was the first to perform bilateral adrenalectomy in patients with prostatic cancer that progressed after orchiectomy [47]. In 1966, Huggins was awarded the Nobel Prize in Physiology or Medicine for his innovative work [48].

Beatson's first bilateral ovariectomy for the treatment of breast cancer was performed without knowledge of the potential carcinogenic effect of female sex hormones. It was the French pathologist Antoine Lacassagne (1884-1971) who showed, 40 years later in 1936, that estrogen administration led to the development of breast cancer in male mice, thus pointing to the relationship between female hormones and the development of breast cancer [49]. In the light of current knowledge, it is interesting to note Lacassagne's intuition of tumor suppressor genes and oncogenes: "It is quite easy to imagine two mechanisms enabling one cell of an organism to liberate itself from subordination to the whole: (a) the loss of something rendering the cell henceforth unable to obey the regulatory inhibitions; (b) the acquisition of something acting as a permanent stimulant [49]". Lacassagne considered hormones to be examples of endogenous stimulation factors. Following Beatson's report, castration by bilateral ovariectomy or irradiation of the ovaries was adopted as a treatment for inoperable, recurrent or metastatic cancer in premenopausal women.

The urine of castrated premenopausal women and of postmenopausal women contains estrogens secreted by the adrenal glands. In 1952, to eliminate this source of estrogens, Charles Huggins removed the adrenals in six women with inoperable and metastatic breast cancer [50]. The same year, removal of the pituitary gland was performed for the same purpose by Herbert Olivecrona (1891-1980), a pioneer of modern neurosurgery [51, 52]. These surgical methods, which yielded similar results but carried a non-negligible morbidity and mortality, were subsequently performed in pre-and postmenopausal women until supplanted by medical hormonal procedures during the 1970s and 1980s. A major problem in surgically removing the ovaries, adrenals or the pituitary gland was the lack of a reliable method to select women with advanced breast cancer who would respond favorably to these procedures, as over fifty per cent of the patients derived no benefit.

At the same time, non-surgical hormonal treatments were being investigated. The use of testosterone propionate, a male hormone, was first reported in 1939 by Alfred Loeser (1889-1963), a British gynecologist, in two cases of breast cancer that recurred within eight months of radical mastectomy and radiation therapy. The medication was given for the treatment of uterine hemorrhages, not for treating the tumor. However, since no further metastases occurred after 18 months, it was inferred that the androgen might have exerted an anti-tumor effect [53]. A clinical trial of synthetic estrogens was also undertaken in the United Kingdom by Alexander Haddow (1907-1970), one of the pioneers of medical oncology [54]. By the early 1950s, the recommendations for first-line treatment of metastatic disease were bilateral ovariectomy in premenopausal women, and estrogens for women five years or more postmenopausal [55]. Androgens were shown to be effective in both pre-and postmenopausal women and mostly used as second-line treatment.

In the mid-sixties, at the time the author began his training in oncology, hormonal treatment whether surgical or medical, was the mainstay against advanced breast cancer. At that time, chemotherapy was offered as a last resort [56].

REFERENCES

[1]   Anonymous. 1. Observations on the antiquity of cancer and metastasis. Cancer Metastasis Rev 2000; 19:193-204.

[2]   Capasso LL. Antiquity of cancer. Int J Cancer 2005; 113:2-13.

[3]   Deeley TJ. A brief history of cancer. Clin Radiol 1983; 34:597-608.

[4]   Rothschild BM, Tanke DH, Helbling M 2nd, Martin LD. Epidemiologic study of tumors in dinosaurs. Naturwissenschaften 2003; 90:495-500.

[5]   Rothschild BM, Witzke BJ, Hershkovitz I. Metastatic cancer in the Jurassic. Lancet 1999; 354:398.

[6]   Nerlich AG, Rohrbach H, Bachmeier B, Zink A. Malignant tumors in two ancient populations: an approach to historical tumor epidemiology. Oncol Rep 2006; 16:197-202.

[7]   Urteaga OB, Pack GT. On the antiquity of melanoma. Cancer 1966; 19:607-10.

[8]   Wells C. Ancient Egyptian pathology. J Laryngol Otol. 1963; 77:261-65.

[9]   Butterfield WC. Tumor treatment, 3000 B.C. Surgery 1966; 60:476-9.

[10]   Littré É. Hippocrate. Oeuvres complètes. Paris: J-B Baillière 1839; Vol II, p 77.

[11]   Ibid. Volume V, p 357.

[12]   Ibid. Volume VI, p 41.

[13]   Shimkin MB. Contrary to Nature. Washington, DC, United States Government Printing Office 1977; DHEW Publication No (NIH) 76-710.

[14]   Hajdu SI. Greco-Roman thought about cancer. Cancer 2004; 100:2048-51.

[15]   Spencer WG. Celsus De Medicina. London: William Heinemann 1935-1938; Vol II, p. 129.

[16]   Reedy J. Galen on cancer and related diseases. Clio Med 1975; 10:227-238.

[17]   Wolff J. Die Lehre von der Krebskrankheit von den ältesten Zeiten bis zur Gegenwart. Volume I; Jena, Gustav Fisher, 1907. English language translation by Barbara Ayoub: The Science of cancerous disease from earliest times to present. Canton, MA, Science History Publications: USA 1989.

[18]   Haddow A. David A. Karnofsky Memorial Lecture. Thoughts on chemical therapy. Cancer 1970; 26:737-54.

[19]   Karpozilos A, Pavlidis N. The treatment of cancer in Greek antiquity. Eur J Cancer 2004; 40:2033-40.

[20]   Hajdu SI, Darvishian F. Diagnosis and treatment of tumors by physicians in antiquity. Ann Clin Lab Sci 2010; 40:386-90.

[21]   Campbell D. Arabian medicine and its influence on the middle ages. London: Kegan Paul, Trench, Trubner & Co 1926; Vol 1, pp. 137-150.

[22]   Osler W. The evolution of modern medicine. New Haven: Yale University Press 1921; pp. 91-104.

[23]   Burns SB, Fulder S. Arabic medicine: preservation and promotion. A millennium of achievement. J Altern Complement Med 2002; 8:407-10.

[24]   Majeed A. How Islam changed medicine. Br Med J 2005; 331:1486-7.

[25]   Smith RD. Avicenna and the Canon of Medicine: A millennial tribute. West J Med 1980; 133:367-70.

[26]   Falagas ME, Zarkadoulia EA, Samonis G. Arab science in the golden age (750-1258 C.E.) and to-day. FASEB 2006; 20:1581-6.

[27]   Al-Fallouji M. Arabs were skilled in anaesthesia. Br Med J 1997; 314:1128.

[28]   Le Dran HF. Mémoire avec un précis de plusieurs observations sur le cancer. Mémoires de l'Académie Royale de Chirugie (Paris) 1715; Tome VII, pp. 223-310.

[29]   Kardinal CG, Yarbro JW. A conceptual history of cancer. Semin Oncol 1979; 6:396-408.

[30]   Ackerknecht EH. Historical notes on cancer. Med Hist 1958; 2:114-9.

[31]   Krumbhaar EB. The centenary of the cell doctrine. Ann Med Hist 1939; 1:427-37.

[32]   Hadju SI. Thoughts about the causes of cancer. Cancer 2006; 106: 1643-9.

[33]   Dumas A. The history of anaesthesia. J Natl Med Assoc 1932; 24:6-9.

[34]   Lister J. On the antiseptic principle in the practice of surgery. Br Med J 1867; 2:246-8.

[35]   On a new kind of rays. By Röntgen WC. Translated by Arthur Stanton from the Sitzungsberichte der Würzburger Physik-medic. Gesellschaft 1895. Nature 1896; 53:274-6.

[36]   Brady LW. Radiation oncology: present status and future potential. CA Cancer J Clin 1976; 26:258-9.

[37]   Beatson GT. On the treatment of inoperable cases of carcinoma of the mamma: suggestions for a new method of treatment with illustrative cases. Lancet 1896; 148:104-7.

[38]   Quimby EH. Historical events leading to the clinical application of radium. CA Cancer J Clin 1966; 16:165-6.

[39]   Pierquin B. Radium therapy from birth to death. 1896-1976. Cancer Radiother 1997; 1:5-13.

[40]   Paul Ehrlich Centennial. Ann NY Acad Sci 1954; 59:143–276.

[41]   Browning CH. Emil Behring and Paul Ehrlich: their contributions to science. Nature 1955; 175:570-75 and 616-19.

[42]   Kasten FH. Paul Ehrlich: pathfinder in cell biology. 1. Chronicle of his life and accomplishments in immunology, cancer research, and chemotherapy. Biotech Histochem 1996; 71:2-37.

[43]   Ehrlich P. Chemotherapeutics: scientific principles, methods, and results. Lancet 1913; 182:445-51.

[44]   Parascandola J. The theoretical basis of Paul Ehrlich's chemotherapy. J Hist Med Allied Sci 1981; 36:19-43.

[45]   Huggins C, Hodges CV. Studies on prostatic cancer: I. The effect of castration, of estrogen and of androgen injection on serum phosphatases in metastatic carcinoma of the prostate. Cancer Res 1941; 1:293-7.

[46]   Huggins C, Stevens RE Jr, Hodges CV. Studies on prostatic cancer. II. The effects of castration on advanced carcinoma of the prostate gland. Arch Surg 1941; 43:209-23.

[47]   Huggins C, Scott WW. Bilateral adrenalectomy in prostatic cancer: clinical features and urinary excretion of 17-ketosteroids and estrogen. Ann Surg 1945; 122:1031-41.

[48]   Huggins C. Endocrine-induced regression of cancers. Cancer Res 1967; 27:1925-30.

[49]   Lacassagne A. Hormonal pathogenesis of adenocarcinoma of the breast. Am J Cancer 1936; 27:217-228.

[50]   Huggins C, Bergenstal DM. Inhibition of human mammary and prostatic cancers by adrenalectomy. Cancer Res 1952; 12:134-41.

[51]   Luft R, Olivecrona H, Sjögren B. Hypophysectomy in man. Nord Med 1952; 47:351-4.

[52]   Machinis TG, Fountas KN. Olivecrona on the development of neurosurgery in the middle of the twentieth century: reflections with the wisdom of today. Neurosurg Focus 2006; 20: E10.

[53]   Loeser AA. Male hormone in the treatment of cancer of the breast. Acta Unio Int Contra Cancrum 1939; 4: 375-6.

[54]   Haddow A, Watkinson JM, Paterson E, Koller PC. Influence of synthetic estrogens on advanced malignant disease. Br Med J 1944; 2:393-8.

[55]   Council on Pharmacy and Chemistry. Current status of hormone therapy of advanced mammary cancer. JAMA 1951; 146: 471-7.

[56]   Green RB, Sethi RS, Lindner HH. Treatment of advanced carcinoma of the breast. Progress in therapy during the past decade. Am J Surg 1964; 108:107-21.

"Cancer chemotherapy had an explosive start". Dr. James Goldie.

"A new fact had been established, however. A chemical compound was at hand which would affect adversely and cause dissolution of a lymphoid neoplasm reputedly resistant to x-rays". Dr. Cornelius P. Rhoads.

CHAPTER 3

World War II's Legacy to Cancer

Pierre R. Band[*]

Department of Medicine, McGill University, Montreal, Canada

Abstract: Medical research carried out during World War II influenced the development of cancer medicine. First, classified research on mustard gas led to the discovery that nitrogen mustard produced tumor regressions in advanced lymphomas. This event marked the dawn of modern cancer chemotherapy. Secondly, the supply of quinine, virtually the sole treatment for malaria, came to a halt after the conquest of Indonesia. As a result, there were more casualties caused by malaria than by combat among American troops fighting in areas where malaria was endemic. To address this critical situation, an extensive cooperative program involving outstanding experimental and clinical investigators was undertaken in the United States to find drugs other than quinine that would be active against malaria. Within a short time, the problem was solved. After the war, several members of the antimalarial program joined the National Institutes of Health. One of them, Dr. Charles Gordon Zubrod, would bring to medical oncology the same vision and organization that made the antimalarial war program a unique success.

Keywords: Mustard gas, mechloretamine, lymphomas, malaria.

FROM CHEMICAL WARFARE TO CANCER TREATMENT

In July 1917, during a battle near Ypres in Belgium, sulfur mustard gas was used for the first time by the Germans, causing many casualties among soldiers and civilians. Mustard gas, also called *yperite* (the name is derived from the name of the Belgian town), is liquid at room temperature and has an odour akin to mustard and garlic. It is a vesicant, producing skin burns and blisters, affecting the respiratory and gastrointestinal tracts and leading to severe bone marrow toxicity with a resulting decrease in white blood cell counts [1]. In a study carried out between the

*Address correspondence to Pierre R. Band: Faculty of Medicine, McGill University, Montreal, Quebec H3G 1Y6, Canada; E-mail: pierre.band@gmail.com

two world wars, the application of solutions of sulfur mustard gas on skin cancers was shown to cause a reduction or disappearance of the treated lesions [2].

I was four years old when World War II broke out. My parents, along with many others, obtained *masques à gaz,* gas masks, to protect us from mustard gas attacks. Luckily, I never had to wear my mask except to play with friends, which, with hindsight, made us all look like ET, the extraterrestrial hero of Steven Spielberg's famous movie produced many years later. Towards the end of the war, the Germans bombed Bari harbor in Italy; ironically, the Allies thought that a major air attack could not occur. A German military reconnaissance plane flew unharmed over the harbor, noticing the Allied ships, including the *SS John Harvey* which carried, in addition to other explosive ammunitions, a secret cargo of about 100 tons of mustard gas bombs. On the evening of December 2, 1943, German planes returned destroying several ships. The *SS John Harvey* exploded, and mustard gas spilled into the sea exposing hundreds of sailors in the oil slick causing severe injuries and death. Colonel Stewart F. Alexander (1914-1991), a consultant in chemical warfare medicine with the Allied Forces Headquarters, was sent to Bari to investigate. Alexander's report contains a detailed description of the clinical findings of mustard gas poisoning, noting that "Individuals did not associate garlic odour and mustard [3]".

Classified wartime research on mustard gas compounds had been carried out in the United States since 1942. Doctors Alfred Gilman (1908-1984) and Louis S. Goodman (1906-2000), known to many medical students around the world for their classic textbook *The Pharmacological Basis of Therapeutics*, studied the pharmacological effects and clinical activity of these compounds at Yale Medical School in New Haven, Connecticut. Their work was published in 1946, after the wartime restriction was lifted. The following observations led to the experimental and clinical evaluation of nitrogen mustards, analogues of the sulfur mustard used as a chemical warfare agent: "The marked effects of the mustards on lymphoid tissue, coupled with the finding that actively proliferating cells are selectively vulnerable to the cytotoxic action of the mustards, suggested the therapeutic use of these compounds in the treatment of neoplasms of lymphoid tissue. Because of its undesirable physical properties and extreme chemical reactivity, sulfur mustard does not lend itself to parenteral administration. However, nitrogen mustard . . . can be readily dissolved in sterile saline for intravenous administration [4]".

The initial clinical investigation of nitrogen mustard followed experimental studies that were never published, but described in a publication twenty years later. Based on the effect of nitrogen mustard on lymphoid tissue, treatment with this compound was initiated in a mouse bearing a transplanted lymphoma; the tumor regressed to the point of no longer being palpable. The study "provided the background for the first clinical trial and indicated the relationship between experimental observations and clinical observations [5]," a relationship that was to become a hallmark of cancer research. The experimental results led to the administration of nitrogen mustard to a patient who was dying from a lymphosarcoma resistant to radiation therapy. The first dose was given in December 1942, one year before the Bari event. Response was dramatic, tumor masses literally melting away; unfortunately, the effect was short-lived and the disease progressed after the third course of therapy. The results of this first clinical trial of nitrogen mustard, which showed therapeutic benefit in patients with Hodgkin's disease, non-Hodgkin's lymphoma and chronic lymphocytic leukemia, not only marked the dawn of modern cancer chemotherapy but also identified one of its major hurdles: drug resistance [6].

These studies initiated by the U.S. Army in preparation for the potential use of chemical agents during World War II, led to a discovery that would benefit mankind instead of being used to destroy it.

The unfolding of these events was related by the U.S. Army Chief of the Medical Division of the Chemical Warfare Service, Dr. Cornelius P. Rhoads (1898-1959), in a publication titled *The sword and the ploughshare* that stands as a classic of modern cancer chemotherapy [7]. Across from United Nations Headquarters in New York City lies a small public park named after American diplomat Ralph Bunche (1903-1971), who won the Nobel Peace Prize in 1950, the first African-American to win that prize. On the wall of the staircase in the park is an inscription from Isaiah 2:4: "They shall beat their swords into plowshares, and their spears into pruning hooks; nation shall not lift up sword against nation, neither shall they learn war any more". That quote inspired the title of Rhoads' publication [8].

Rhoads was a visionary, an inspiring and captivating person who had a dream: developing a cancer oriented research center. Together with Frank

Howard an associate of Mr. Alfred Sloan, he convinced Alfred Sloan and Charles Kettering, former General Motors executives, to fund a new basic and clinical cancer research center, the Sloan-Kettering Institute for Cancer Research. There was more to this story. Rhoads had a missing finger; it was amputated in the late thirties because of a severe infection. The infection spread to his arm and his life was endangered. The Chairman of Medicine at Yale University at the time had just returned from a sabbatical in Europe with an interesting new compound called sulfanilamide. That saved Rhoads' arm and probably his life, and likely reinforced, or may have initiated his belief that if you could cure an infection with a chemical you ought to be able to cure cancer with one [8].

FROM METHYLENE BLUE TO ONCOLOGY

Malaria, the disease caused by the parasite called *Plasmodium*, is transmitted to human through the bite of an infected mosquito. The number of affected cases in 2009, estimated by the World Health Organization, was 225 million, with about three quarters of a million deaths, 85% of them children under five years of age [9]. In the 17th century, Jesuits introduced the bark of the cinchona tree, from which quinine is extracted, from South America into Europe. Until the mid-forties, quinine remained virtually the sole treatment for malaria, and supply depended on the availability of the cinchona bark. Over 90% of the cinchona trees come from plantations on the island of Java in Indonesia, which at the time of World War II was part of the Dutch East Indies.

Ehrlich showed that methylene blue stained the malaria parasite. As methylene blue is virtually non-toxic, would it not act as a "magic bullet" against malaria? Indeed, in 1891, methylene blue was given to two patients with acute febrile episodes of malaria (Fig. **3.1**): the fever abated and the parasites disappeared from the blood of these patients [10]. That event is considered the beginning of modern chemotherapy.

This observation served as a lead for chemists at Eberfeld Laboratories of the Bayer I.G. Farbenindustrie in Germany to synthesize two active antimalarial drugs, quinacrine and resorchin, before World War II. These compounds, however, were considered too toxic and did not replace quinine as the standard medication for treating malaria.

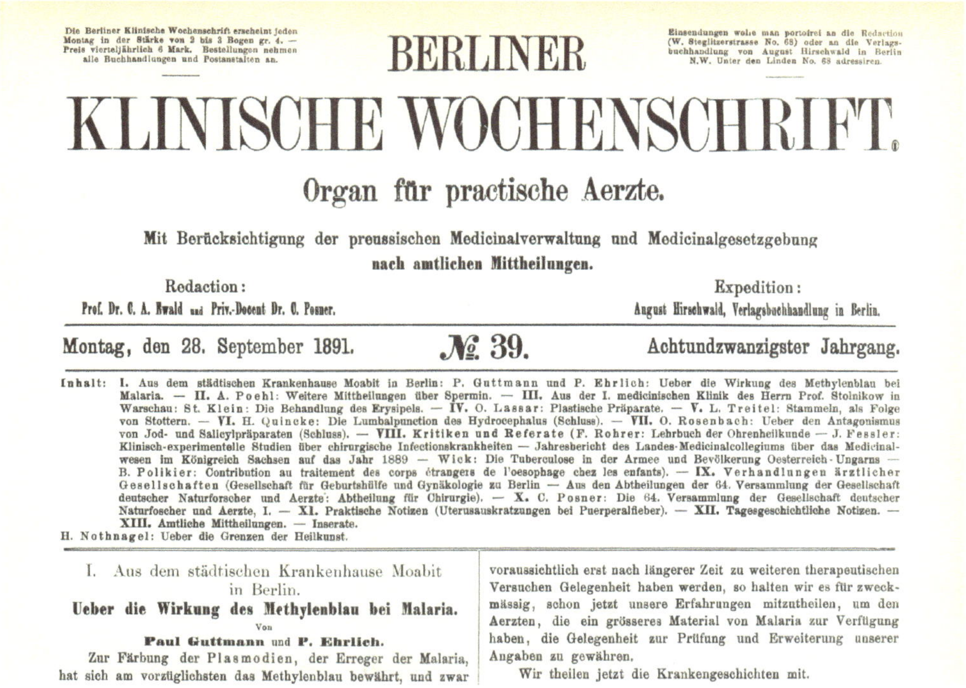

Die Berliner Klinische Wochenschrift erscheint jeden Montag in der Stärke von 2 bis 3 Bogen gr. 4. — Preis vierteljährlich 6 Mark. Bestellungen nehmen alle Buchhandlungen und Postanstalten an.

Einsendungen wolle man portofrei an die Redaction (W. Steglitzerstrasse No. 68) oder an die Verlagsbuchhandlung von August Hirschwald in Berlin N.W. Unter den Linden No. 68 adressiren.

BERLINER

KLINISCHE WOCHENSCHRIFT.

Organ für practische Aerzte.

Mit Berücksichtigung der preussischen Medicinalverwaltung und Medicinalgesetzgebung nach amtlichen Mittheilungen.

Redaction: Prof. Dr. C. A. Ewald und Priv.-Docent Dr. C. Posner.

Expedition: August Hirschwald, Verlagsbuchhandlung in Berlin.

Montag, den 28. September 1891. № 39. Achtundzwanzigster Jahrgang.

Inhalt: I. Aus dem städtischen Krankenhause Moabit in Berlin: P. Guttmann und P. Ehrlich: Ueber die Wirkung des Methylenblau bei Malaria. — II. A. Poehl: Weitere Mittheilungen über Spermin. — III. Aus der I. medicinischen Klinik des Herrn Prof. Stolnikow in Warschau: St. Klein: Die Behandlung des Erysipels. — IV. O. Lassar: Plastische Präparate. — V. L. Treitel: Stammeln, als Folge von Stottern. — VI. H. Quincke: Die Lumbalpunction des Hydrocephalus (Schluss). — VII. O. Rosenbach: Ueber den Antagonismus von Jod- und Salicylpräparaten (Schluss). — VIII. Kritiken und Referate (F. Rohrer: Lehrbuch der Ohrenheilkunde — J. Fessler: Klinisch-experimentelle Studien über chirurgische Infectionskrankheiten — Jahresbericht des Landes-Medicinalcollegiums über das Medicinalwesen im Königreich Sachsen auf das Jahr 1889 — Wick: Die Tuberculose in der Armee und Bevölkerung Oesterreich-Ungarns — B. Polikier: Contribution au traitement des corps étrangers de l'oesophage chez les enfants). — IX. Verhandlungen ärztlicher Gesellschaften (Gesellschaft für Geburtshülfe und Gynäkologie zu Berlin — Aus den Abtheilungen der 64. Versammlung der Gesellschaft deutscher Naturforscher und Aerzte: Abtheilung für Chirurgie). — X. C. Posner: Die 64. Versammlung der Gesellschaft deutscher Naturfoscher und Aerzte, I. — XI. Praktische Notizen (Uterusauskratzungen bei Puerperalfieber). — XII. Tagesgeschichtliche Notizen. — XIII. Amtliche Mittheilungen. — Inserate.
H. Nothnagel: Ueber die Grenzen der Heilkunst.

I. Aus dem städtischen Krankenhause Moabit in Berlin.

Ueber die Wirkung des Methylenblau bei Malaria.

Von

Paul Guttmann und **P. Ehrlich.**

Zur Färbung der Plasmodien, der Erreger der Malaria, hat sich am vorzüglichsten das Methylenblau bewährt, und zwar voraussichtlich erst nach längerer Zeit zu weiteren therapeutischen Versuchen Gelegenheit haben werden, so halten wir es für zweckmässig, schon jetzt unsere Erfahrungen mitzutheilen, um den Aerzten, die ein grösseres Material von Malaria zur Verfügung haben, die Gelegenheit zur Prüfung und Erweiterung unserer Angaben zu gewähren.

Wir theilen jetzt die Krankengeschichten mit.

Figure 3.1: The treatment of malaria with methylene blue: Ehrlich's first chemotherapeutic study was based on experimental evidence demonstrating the uptake of methylene blue by the malaria parasite. Reproduced from Berl Klin Wochenschrift 1891; 39: 953-6, reference 10.

During World War II, after Holland and Indonesia were conquered by the Germans and the Japanese respectively, the supply of quinine to the United States came to a halt at a time when American troops and Marines were fighting in areas where malaria was endemic or hyper-endemic. The two *Plasmodium* species to which soldiers were exposed were *Plamodium falciparum* and *Plasmodium vivax*, the former causing the most common form of malaria. There were more casualties caused by malaria than by combat with the Japanese, a situation aptly described by General Douglas MacArthur (1880-1964): "This will be a long war if for every division I have facing the enemy I must count on a second division in hospital with malaria and a third division convalescing from this debilitating disease [11]". In response to this critical situation, the United States undertook an extensive cooperative program against malaria, involving government, academia and the pharmaceutical industry.

The objectives were first to find appropriate and available drugs other than quinine that could be used to prevent malaria, suppress its clinical symptoms and potentially cure the disease, and secondly, to develop new compounds [12]. The chairman of the Clinical Testing Panel of the Board for the Coordination of Malarial Studies, Dr. James Shannon (1904-1994), surrounded himself with outstanding scientists and innovators, including Dr. Julius Axelrod (1912-2004), a future Nobel Prize recipient. This research group, often referred to as the Goldwater antimalarial group because their work took place at Goldwater Memorial Hospital on Welfare Island in the East River across from Manhattan, tackled the first objective [13]. The chosen drug was quinacrine, but the recommended dosage had not been based on sound pharmacological methods and it produced side effects, resulting in poor compliance. First, an analytical method was developed to accurately measure levels of quinacrine in the blood, other fluids and tissues. Using this assay, the pharmacology and toxicology of quinacrine were studied in experimental animal systems and in humans. Drug dosage was correlated with blood concentrations and therapeutic effect in humans with *falciparum* and *vivax* malaria in order to derive a recommended dosage that would be both active and relatively well tolerated. Within a year, quinacrine was established and considered superior to quinine for suppressing symptoms and curing *falciparum* malaria and in suppressing symptoms but not curing *vivax* malaria. The use of quinacrine in the United States Army and Navy resulted in a dramatic reduction of casualties from malaria [11]. In addition, a national cooperative effort involving screening of several compounds in avian malarias, as well as experimental pharmacological and clinical investigations, led to the rediscovery of chloroquine which was shown to be superior to quinacrine in the treatment of *vivax* malaria. Indeed, chloroquine was found to be similar to resorchin, the antimalaria drug previously synthesized by Bayer scientists, but overlooked in terms of its therapeutic value [14].

The malarial war program was a gigantic cooperative effort, focussing on one disease and involving a number of disciplines and techniques, including chemistry, drug screening in experimental animal systems, experimental and human pharmacology and toxicology and clinical trials. After the war, Shannon became director of the National Institutes of Health, and several key Goldwater antimalarial research group members also joined this organization. One of them would bring to medical oncology the same vision and organization that had made the antimalarial war program a unique success. His name was Dr. Charles Gordon Zubrod.

The end of the first half of the 20th century also witnessed the introduction, under the leadership of Sir Bradford Hill (1897-1991), of the controlled clinical trial using individual random assignment [15]. This innovative approach was to become an essential part of cancer medicine, not only as a tool for drug evaluation, but as a new way of practice to investigate research questions [16].

REFERENCES

[1]   Krumbhaar EB, Krumbhaar HD. The blood and bone marrow in yellow cross gas (mustard gas) poisoning: changes produced in the bone marrow of fatal cases. J Med Res 1919; 40:497-508.

[2]   Adair FE, Bagg HJ. Experimental and clinical studies on the treatment of cancer by dichloroethylsulphide (mustard gas). Ann Surg 1931; 93:190-9.

[3]   Alexander SF. Medical report of the Bari harbor mustard casualties. Mil Surg 1947; 101:1-17.

[4]   Gilman A, Philips FS. The biological actions and therapeutic applications of the B-chloroethyl amines and sulfides. Science 1946; 103:409-15 and 436.

[5]   Gilman A. The initial clinical trial of nitrogen mustard. Am J Surg 1963; 105:574-8.

[6]   Goodman LS, Wintrobe MM, Dameshek W, Goodman MJ, Gilman A, McLennan MT. Nitrogen mustard therapy; use of methyl-bis (beta-chloroethyl) amine hydrochloride and tris (beta-chloroethyl) amine hydrochloride for Hodgkin's disease, lymphosarcoma, leukemia and certain allied and miscellaneous disorders. JAMA 1946; 132:126-32.

[7]   Rhoads CP. The sword and the ploughshare. J Mt Sinai Hosp 1946; 13:299-309.

[8]   Author's interview with Dr. Irwin H. Krakoff, July 2011.

[9]   World Health Organization. World Malaria Report 2010.

[10]   Guttman P, Ehrlich P. Ueber die Wirkung des Methylenblau bei Malaria. Berl Klin Wochenschrift 1891; 39:953-6.

[11]   Condon-Rall ME. Allied cooperation in malaria prevention and control: the World War II Southwest Pacific experience. J Hist Med Allied Sci 1991; 46:493-513.

[12]   Shannon JA. Chemotherapy in malaria. Bull NY Acad Med 1946; 22:345-57.

[13]   Shannon JA. The study of antimalarials and antimalarial activity in the human malarias. Harvey Lect 1945-1946; 41:43-89.

[14]   Coatney GR. Pitfalls in a discovery: the chronicle of chloroquine. Am J Trop Med Hyg 1963; 12:121-8.

[15]   Streptomycin treatment of pulmonary tuberculosis: a Medical Research Council investigation. Br Med J 1948; 2:769-82.

[16]   Keating P, Cambrosio A. Cancer clinical trials: the emergence and development of a new style of practice. Bull Hist Med 2007; 81:197-223.

"Sound scientific endeavour and fortitude can find answers to the most complicated and discouraging problem." Dr. Edward C. Kendall.

CHAPTER 4

The Immediate Post-World War II Years: Cancer Chemotherapy Spreads its Wings

Pierre R. Band[*]

Department of Medicine, McGill University, Montreal, Canada

Abstract: Dr. Lucy Wills, a British hematologist, worked in India on "pernicious anemia of pregnancy" which was later found to be caused by folic acid deficiency. Dr. Yellapragada Subbarow synthesized that vitamin, as well as analogues that blocked its activities, including the drugs aminopterin and methotrexate. Aminopterin, first used by Dr. Sidney Farber, induced complete remissions in children with acute lymphocytic leukemia. Dr. Cornelius P. Rhoads was the U.S. Army Chief of the Medical Division of the Chemical Warfare Service during World War II. When the war ended, an outstanding group of scientists and clinicians who had served under him went on to play a major role in the development of medical oncology. Three of them, Doctors David Karnofsky, Frederick Philips, and Chester C. Stock, as well as Dr. Joseph H. Burchenal, joined Rhoads at the Memorial Hospital and Sloan-Kettering Institute for Cancer Research. The Memorial group developed a broad-scope cancer chemotherapy program that included screening, pharmacology, clinical investigation of chemotherapeutic agents and liaison with the pharmaceutical industry. During those years, two other important anticancer drugs were synthesized: cortisone by Dr. Edward C. Kendall and Tadeusz Reichstein, and 6-mercaptopurine by Doctors George H. Hitchings and Gertrude B. Elion. These scientists received the Nobel Prize in Physiology or Medicine for their achievements

Keywords: Aminopterin, methotrexate, cortisone, 6-mercaptopurine.

BOSTON CHILDREN'S HOSPTAL

Dr. Lucy Wills (1888-1964), a British hematologist, worked in India on "pernicious anemia of pregnancy". The illness was often fatal among poor and malnourished pregnant Indian women, few remaining in hospital to receive treatment: "if a woman can crawl she must attend to her home duties [1]". Wills

---

*Address correspondence to Pierre R. Band:** Faculty of Medicine, McGill University, Montreal, Quebec H3G 1Y6, Canada; E-mail: pierre.band@gmail.com

showed that this anemia differed from true pernicious anemia and could be cured by crude liver extract and by Marmite, a British food spread made from brewer's yeast. She suggested that "some deficiency in the vitamin B complex was significant as a causative factor" and recommended Marmite for its "advantage in India of being comparatively cheap and of vegetable origin [1]". The factor, present in liver and yeast and particularly in green vegetables, was extracted and highly concentrated in "probably nearly pure form" from four tons of spinach; it was named folic acid from the Latin word *folium* meaning leaf [2]. Subsequent work by a group of investigators under the leadership of a brilliant Indian biochemist, Dr. Yellapragada Subbarow (1895-1948) at Lederle Laboratories with colleagues at Calco Chemical Division, American Cyanamide Company, led to the synthesis of pteroylglutamic acid, the chemical name for folic acid, and of folic acid congeners [3].

Around the same time, a group of researchers at Mount Sinai Hospital in New York City reported that fresh brewer's yeast induced complete regression of spontaneous mammary tumors in mice [4]. A similar effect was noted with a folic acid congener later known as pteroyltriglutamic acid [5]. Based on these data, Dr. Sidney Farber (1903-1973) treated various hematologic malignancies and advanced solid tumors with pteroyltriglutamic acid and polyglutamate congeners (diopterin and teropterin) with some possible benefit [6]. The legendary American baseball hero Babe Ruth was treated by others with teropterin, which gave it currency. Subbarow's group had also synthesized several analogues, including aminopterin, which blocked folic acid activities *in vitro* and in mice [7]. In a landmark article published in June 1948 in the *New England Journal of Medicine*, Farber at the Children's Hospital in Boston (Fig. **4.1**) reported marked improvement and a complete remission with aminopterin in five children with acute lymphocytic leukemia, four of whom were critically ill before the start of therapy [8]. Soon afterwards, another folic acid antagonist, methotrexate (amethopterin) with a better therapeutic index in mice, also obtained from Subbarow, was shown to be effective against childhood acute leukemia and supplanted aminopterin in the treatment of that disease.

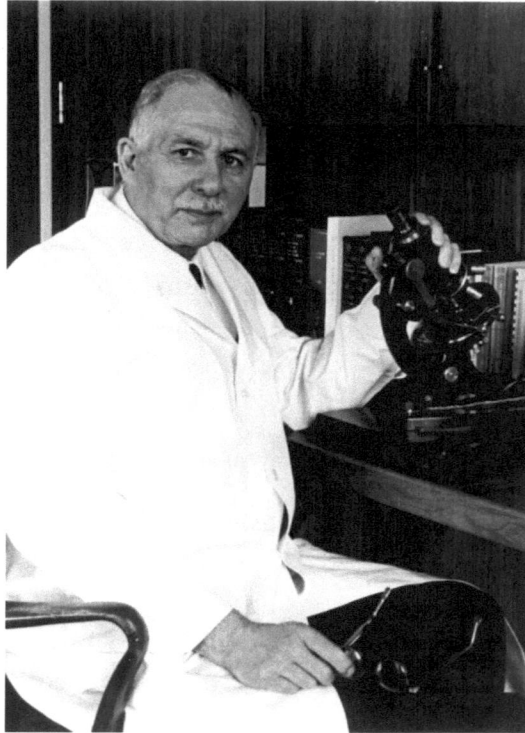

Figure 4.1: Dr. Sidney Farber. Courtesy of the Dana-Farber Cancer Institute.

Farber remained an innovator in medical oncology, exerting considerable influence. His opinion was widely sought and valued. He also collaborated with Mary Lasker (1900-1994), who led the effort in the development of the Cancer Chemotherapy National Service Center, and played a major role in the political and scientific events that led to the National Cancer Act in the United States.

As previously mentioned, Mathé was Head of the Hematology Department at the Institut Gustave-Roussy. Many children from all over Europe who were suffering from acute leukemia were referred to Mathé's department for treatment. While I was there, I happened to take care of a critically ill Hungarian girl who was eight years old. She died soon after admission, white, with blood on her lips. Her father, a physician who didn't realize I understood Hungarian, bent over, kissed her on the forehead and said: "What will I tell your mother?" All of us who trained in cancer medicine at that time had similar painful experiences. It is difficult for anyone who didn't live the days when childhood acute leukemia was a dreadfully rapid and fatal illness to fully grasp the tremendous scientific and emotional impact of Farber's breakthrough. For the first time, the hope of curing human cancer with medication became a real possibility.

MEMORIAL HOSPITAL AND SLOAN-KETTERING INSTITUTE FOR CANCER RESEARCH

In January 1940, Dr. Cornelius P. Rhoads (1898-1959), a pathologist, was appointed Scientific Director of the Memorial Hospital in New York City; he later became Director of the Sloan-Kettering Institute for Cancer Research. "The announcement of the opening of the Institute scheduled for August 8, 1945, happened two days after the atomic bomb was dropped on Hiroshima; consequently, it received little media publicity [9]". In 1960, the hospital and institute became one, the Memorial Sloan-Kettering Cancer Center. Memorial Hospital was one of the world's oldest hospitals devoted to the treatment of cancer patients, being mainly at that time a center for surgery and radiation therapy. During World War II, Rhoads was the U.S. Army Chief of the Medical Division of the Chemical Warfare Service. An outstanding group of clinicians and scientists who were destined to play a major role in the development of medical oncology served under him: Doctors David Karnofsky (1914-1969), Frederick Philips (1916-1984), Howard Skipper (1915-2006) and Chester C. Stock (1910-2008).

After the war, all of them except Skipper joined Rhoads at Memorial Hospital (Fig. **4.2**). Skipper went to the Southern Research Institute in Birmingham, Alabama, where he led an experimental research program that would greatly influence the therapy of malignant diseases. After being discharged from the military, Dr. Joseph H. Burchenal (1912-2006) returned to Memorial Hospital where he had begun his career.

At the Sloan-Kettering Institute for Cancer Research, Rhoads structured a broad-scope cancer chemotherapy program that included screening, toxicology, pharmacology and clinical investigation of chemotherapeutic agents. He also established liaison with the pharmaceutical industry. "He would go to drug companies and say 'you have interesting chemicals, let us test them in animals and see what could result'; he built this whole working relationship with the pharmaceutical industry [9]". Stock headed the Division of Experimental Chemotherapy, aimed at discovering compounds with selective antitumor effects. A large number of agents were tested, mainly using the transplanted mouse Sarcoma 180 as a primary screen [10, 11]. Philips, who had worked in the laboratory of Doctors Goodman and Gilman at Yale Medical School on the biological action of nitrogen and sulfur mustards, became Head of the Pharmacology Section of the Division of Experimental Chemotherapy. During his career, Philips studied the pre-clinical pharmacology and toxicology of many important cancer chemotherapeutic drugs [12].

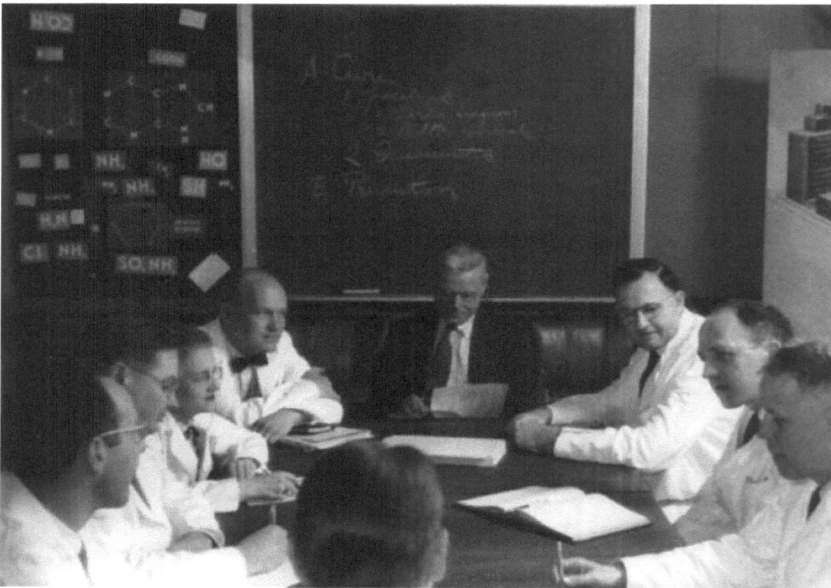

Figure 4.2: From left to right: Doctors Frederick Philips, John Biesele, Christine Reilly, Joseph H. Burchenal, Cornelius Rhoads, Chester C. Stock, David Karnofsky, George Wooley. Photograph taken by Ike Vern, circa 1956. Courtesy of the Memorial Sloan-Kettering Cancer Center.

Burchenal and Karnofsky were primarily clinical investigators. Together, they formed the most prominent creative and visionary team of physicians in the early effort against cancer. It is impossible to do justice to their contributions individually, as the two usually co-authored important publications. Karnofsky died of lung cancer, possibly related to mustard gas exposure. As Burchenal wrote: "During the planning of a field trial in which a small number of goats were to be subjected to mustard gas, Dave, a first lieutenant, suggested that more significant data might be obtained using several hundred mice placed at strategic intervals instead of a few goats. When the colonel in charge replied that mice were too small and goats, being larger, were naturally much better, Dave proposed that perhaps one should carry this theory further by dispensing with the goats entirely and using one elephant instead [13]". Two days later he was sent to a camp in Florida "where he spent months tethering goats in appropriate locations . . . After the plane with the mustard gas had finished spraying . . . he often carried the intoxicated goats out of the testing area himself [13]". To this, Dr. Irwin Krakoff, a long time friend and colleague of Karnofsky, added: "Regardless of that he had a lot of exposure to nitrogen mustard and had mustard burns on his hands [9]".

Karnofsky, who participated in the early experimental and clinical investigation of nitrogen mustard, had a profound knowledge of tumor biology and cancer medicine. In 1948, he discussed the various facets of cancer chemotherapy in the *New England Journal of Medicine* [14-16] and developed criteria for the clinical evaluation of chemotherapeutic agents [17, 18]: "It is necessary, therefore, to examine, from the clinician's point of view, the problem of evaluating chemotherapeutic agents against cancer, and to arrive at some criteria whereby we can determine the therapeutic activity of, and indications for, the use of a new agent [17]". Karnofsky's performance status categories, described in 1949 and still used today [17], are based on an astute clinical observation: "The fact that subjective and objective evidence of improvement can occur in a patient, while the patient continues to remain bedridden, has suggested to us the need for another criterion of effect. This has been called the performance status or PS [17]". In 1955, Karnofsky initiated a useful review of chemotherapeutic agents (Fig. **4.3**) that was periodically revised [19]. After Karnofsky's death, the reviews were updated by Krakoff.

CORTISONE

"The preparation of cholesterol, cortisone and hydrocortisone by total synthesis will always remain as landmarks of organic chemistry [20]". One thousand kilograms of cattle adrenal glands were needed to produce the 25 grams of concentrated extracts from which one of 29 steroids, compound E, later called

SPECIFIC AGENTS USED IN CANCER CHEMOTHERAPY

AGENTS	PRINCIPAL ROUTE OF ADMINIST.	USUAL DOSE	ACUTE TOXIC SIGNS	MAJOR LATE TOXIC MANIFESTATIONS
POLYFUNCTIONAL ALKYLATING AGENTS				
Methylbis(β-chloroethyl)amine HCl (HN2) Mustargen®	I.V.	0.4 mg./Kg. single or divided doses	N. & V.*	Therapeutic doses moderately depress peripheral blood-cell count; excessive doses cause severe bone-marrow depression with leukopenia, thrombocytopenia, and bleeding. Maximum toxicity may occur two or three weeks after last dose. Dosage, therefore, must be carefully controlled.
p-carboxylpropylphenylbis-(β-chloroethyl)amine (CB1348)	Oral	4-8 mg. daily	None	
Triethylenemelamine TEM®	I.V. Oral	0.04 mg./Kg. x 3 20-40 mg. in 1 mo.	Occasional N. & V.*	
triethylenephosphoramide (TEPA)	I.M.	0.2 mg./Kg. x 5	None	
triethylenethiophosphoramide (ThioTEPA)	Oral I.V.	5-10 mg./day 0.2 mg./Kg. x 5	None	
1,4-Dimethanesulfonyloxybutane (GT-41) Myleran®	Oral	2-8 mg./day 150-250 mg./course	None	
ANTIMETABOLITES				
4-Amino-N¹⁰-methylpteroylglutamic acid (Amethopterin) Methotrexate®	Oral	2.5-5.0 mg./day	None	Oral and digestive-tract ulcerations; bone-marrow depression with leukopenia, thrombocytopenia, and bleeding.
4-Aminopteroylglutamic acid (Aminopterin)	Oral	0.25-1.0 mg./day		
6-Mercaptopurine (6-MP) Purinethol®	Oral	2.5 mg./Kg./day	None	Therapeutic doses usually well tolerated; excessive doses cause bone-marrow depression.
6-thioguanine (6-TG)	Oral	2.5 mg./Kg./day		
6-chloropurine (6-CP)	Oral	20 mg./Kg./day		
Azaserine Serynl®	Oral	2.5 mg./Kg./day (with 6-MP)	None	Sore, red tongue.
STEROID HORMONES				
Androgen Testosterone propionate	I.M.	50-100 mg. 3 x weekly	None	Fluid retention, masculinization.
Methyltestosterone	Oral	100 mg. daily		
Estrogen Diethylstilbestrol	Oral	1-5 mg. 3 x daily	Occasional N. & V.*	Fluid retention, feminization, uterine bleeding.
Ethinyl estradiol	Oral	0.1-1.0 mg. 3 x daily		
Adrenal Cortical Hormones Cortisone® acetate	Oral	50-300 mg. daily	None	Fluid retention, hypertension, diabetes, increased susceptibility to infection.
Hydrocortisone acetate	Oral	50-200 mg. daily		
Meticorten®	Oral	20-100 mg. daily		
Adrenocorticotropic Hormone (ACTH)	I.V. I.M.	25-50 mg. by continuous infusion 10-20 mg. every 3 hr.	None	
RADIOACTIVE ISOTOPES				
Iodine (I¹³¹)	Oral, I.V.	100-200 mc.	None	Myxedema, bone-marrow depression, renal damage.
Phosphorus (P³²)	Oral, I.V.	3-7 mc.	None	Bone-marrow depression
Gold (Au¹⁹⁸)	Intrapleur. Intra-abd.	75 mc. 75 mc.	None	Bone-marrow depression.
MISCELLANEOUS DRUGS				
Urethane	Oral	2-4 gm. daily	N. & V.*	Bone-marrow depression.
Potassium arsenite (Fowler's solution)	Oral	0.2-1 cc. daily	None	Diarrhea, vomiting, skin eruptions.

*N. & V. = Nausea and vomiting

Figure 4.3: Page 170 in: Karnofsky DA. Chemotherapy of cancer. CA Cancer J Clin 1955; 5:165-73, reference 19. Reproduced with permission from John Wiley and Sons.

cortisone, was isolated [21]. In 1950, Dr. Edward C. Kendall (1886-1972) and Philip S. Hench (1896-1965) from the Mayo Clinic in Rochester, Minnesota, and Dr. Tadeusz Reichstein (1891-1996), a Polish born doctor working at Basel University in Switzerland, shared the Nobel Prize in Physiology or Medicine for its discovery. Collaboration between the pharmaceutical firm Merck and Company, Inc., New Jersey, and Kendall's laboratory led to large-scale production of cortisone for clinical trials.

An amusing story may have given impetus to the synthesis of steroid hormones in the United States. "Attention focused on a rumor that Germany was buying beef adrenal glands in South America for the purpose of making adrenal cortical extract. It was said the extract was being used to counteract the hypoxia of Luftwaffe pilots to permit them to fly at higher altitude . . . The Medical Research Division of the Office of Scientific Research and Development gave top priority to the synthesis of Kendall's Compound A [22]". The project was abandoned as Compound A did not meet expectations. However, Kendall and his group continued their research on the isolation of adrenal steroids. It is said that the medication taken by the Nazi pilots was called "Göring pills" [23] after the Commander-in-Chief of the Luftwaffe during World War II.

The fact that cortisone and adrenocorticotropin hormone produced involution of lymphoid tissue suggested the potential use of cortisone in experimental murine lymphosarcoma and leukemia, resulting in tumor regression and increased survival respectively [24, 25]. In 1948, Dr. Olof H. Pearson (1913-1990) and colleagues at Memorial Hospital were the first to initiate clinical studies of cortisone in lymphomas and leukemias. Shrinkage of tumor masses was observed in lymphomas, with good clinical and hematologic responses in acute leukemia. Of substantial interest, a lack of cross-resistance with folic acid antagonists was noted [26, 27]; subsequently, a lack of cross-resistance with 6-mercaptopurine was also reported [28].

6-MERCAPTOPURINE

The drug 6-mercaptopurine was, with aminopterin, the first cancer chemotherapeutic agent synthesized with a biochemical rationale. Its development from synthesis to experimental and clinical investigation was the fruit of a collaborative endeavour between the pharmaceutical industry and the Sloan-Kettering Institute for Cancer Research. Dr. George H. Hitchings (1905-1998) began his career at Burroughs Wellcome Research Laboratories in Tuckahoe, New York, as the sole member of the Biochemistry Department, later joined by Dr. Gertrude B. Elion (1918-1999). They shared the Nobel Prize in Physiology or Medicine in 1988 for their work on purine and pyrimidine analogues. In her Nobel Prize lecture, Elion related the theoretical bases and events leading to the synthesis of 6-mercaptopurine after more than 100 purines had been tested [29]. In his Nobel Prize lecture, Hitchings said: "Now we have the chemotherapeutic agents; we need only to find the diseases [30]". Burchenal would provide the answer. The compound 6-mercaptopurine, found to inhibit the growth of the experimental Sarcoma 180 tumor [31], was studied in patients suffering from various malignancies. In a landmark publication, Burchenal reported that 15 of 45 children with acute lymphocytic leukemia developed complete hematologic and clinical remissions with partial remissions occurring in ten other children [28]. Furthermore, remissions were obtained in some patients who had been resistant to previous treatment with methotrexate.

Reminiscing about those times, Krakoff (Fig 4.4), who joined the Memorial Hospital in 1953 and later became chief of the Medical Oncology Service at Memorial Hospital and Chief of the Division of Chemotherapy at the Sloan-Kettering Institute for Cancer Research, concluded:

> Burchenal and Karnofsky were totally different people in personality. Karnofsky was methodical, taking a systematic look at things, whereas Burchenal was more compulsive and less organized; for example, Burchenal was studying mouse leukemia and had a colony of mice in his garage! However, they complemented each other very well and formed a good team. In my mind, Karnofsky is the father of us all; he instilled methods and thoughtfulness in cancer medicine, made it respectable and scientifically credible. He was the major factor to legitimize cancer medicine. Between 1946 and 1953, The Sloan-Kettering Institute paved the way for pre-clinical and clinical cancer research activities [9].

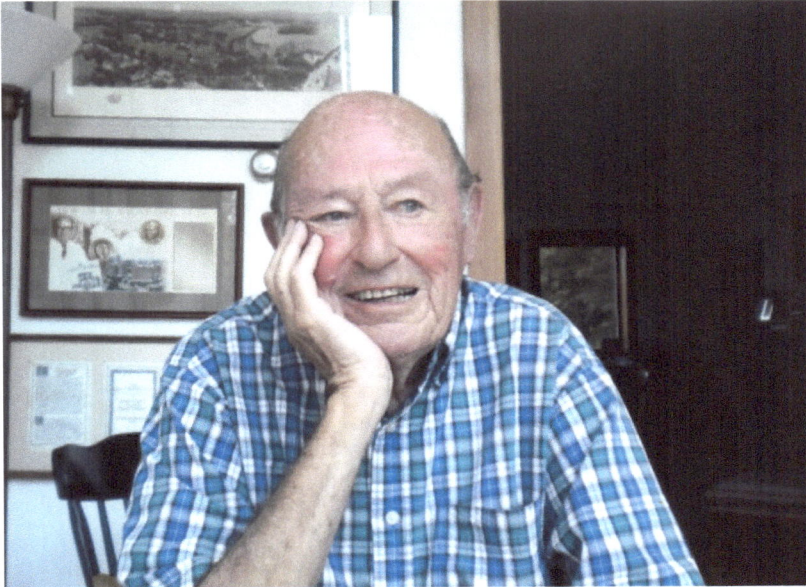

Figure 4.4: Dr. Irwin H. Krakoff. Photo taken by the author, July 2011.

And so, by 1953, three non-cross resistant drugs, methotrexate, cortisone and 6-mercaptopurine, had been shown to be active, most effectively against childhood acute leukemia. That same year saw the opening in Bethesda, Maryland, of the U.S. National Institutes of Health Clinical Center, a hospital devoted to clinical research.

REFERENCES

[1]   Wills L. Treatment of "pernicious anaemia of pregnancy" and "tropical anemia". Br Med J 1931; 1:1059-64.

[2]   Mitchell HK, Snell EE, Williams RJ. The concentration of "folic acid ". J Am Chem Soc 1941; 63:2284 (Letter).

[3]   Folic Acid. Ann NY Acad Sci 1946; 48:257-350.

[4]   Lewisohn R, Leuchtenberger C, Leuchtenberger R, Laszlo D. The treatment of spontaneous breast adenocarcinoma in mice with extracts of spleen or yeast. Am J Pathol 1941; 17:251-60.

[5]   Lewisohn R, Leuchtenberger C, Leuchtenberger R, Keresztesy JC. The influence of liver *L casei* factor on spontaneous breast cancer in mice. Science 1946; 104:436-7.

[6]   Farber S, Cutler EC, Hawkins JW, Harrison JH, Peirce EC 2nd, Lenz GG. The action of pteroylglutamic conjugates on man. Science 1947; 106:619-21.

[7]   Oleson JJ, Hutchings BL, Subbarow Y. Studies on the inhibitory nature of 4-aminopteroylglutamic acid. J Biol Chem 1948; 175:359-65.

[8]   Farber S, Diamond LK, Mercer RD, Sylvester RF Jr, Wolff JA. Temporary remissions in acute leukemia in children produced by folic acid antagonist, 4-aminopteroyl-glutamic acid (aminopterin). N Engl J Med 1948; 238:787-93.

[9]   Author's interview with Dr. Irwin H. Krakoff.

[10]   Stock CC. Aspects of approaches in experimental cancer chemotherapy. Am J Med 1950; 8:658-74.

[11]   Stock CC. Experimental cancer chemotherapy. Adv Cancer Res 1954; 2:425-92.

[12]   Stock CC. Obituary: Frederick S. Philips 1916-1984. Cancer Res 1984; 44:3639-40.

[13]   Burchenal JH. Obituary: David A. Karnofsky. Cancer Res 1970; 30:549-50.

[14]   Karnofsky DA. Chemotherapy of neoplastic disease; methods of approach. N Engl J Med 1948; 239:226-31.

[15]   Karnofsky DA. Chemotherapy of neoplastic disease; trends in experimental cancer therapy. N Engl J Med 1948; 239:260-70.

[16]   Karnofsky DA. Chemotherapy of neoplastic disease: agents of clinical value. N Engl J Med 1948; 239:299-305.

[17]   Karnofsky DA, Burchenal JH. The clinical evaluation of chemotherapeutic agents in cancer. New York: Columbia University Press 1949; pp. 191-205.

[18]   Karnofsky DA. Meaningful clinical classification of therapeutic responses to anticancer drugs. Clin Pharmacol Ther 1961; 2:709-12.

[19]   Karnofsky DA. Chemotherapy of cancer. CA Cancer J Clin 1955; 5:165-173.

[20]   Kendall EC. Hormones of the adrenal cortex. Bull NY Acad Med 1953; 29:91-100.

[21]   Reichstein T. Chemistry of the adrenal cortex hormones. Nobel lecture (Physiology or Medicine), December 11, 1950. Amsterdam: Elsevier 1962; pp. 291-307.

[22]   Ingle DJ. Dr. Edward C. Kendall. Biogr Mem Natl Acad Sci 1974; 47:249-90.

[23]   Pasero G, Marson P. A short history of anti-rheumatic therapy. IV. Corticosteroids. Reumatismo 2010; 62:292-9.

[24]   Heilman FR, Kendall EC. The influence of 11-dehydro-17-hydroxycorticosterone (compound E) on the growth of a malignant tumor in the mouse. Endocrinology 1944; 34:416-20.

[25]   Murphy JB, Sturm E. The effect of adrenal cortical and pituitary adrenotropic hormones on transplanted leukemia in rats. Science; 1944; 99:303.

[26]   Pearson OH, Eliel LP, Rawson RW, Dobriner K, Rhoads CP. ACTH-and cortisone -induced regression of lymphoid tumors in man. A preliminary report. Cancer 1949; 2:943-5.

[27]   Pearson OH, Eliel LP. Use of pituitary adrenocorticotropic hormone (ACTH) and cortisone in lymphomas and leukemias. JAMA 1950; 144:1349-53.

[28]   Burchenal JH, Murphy ML, Ellison RR, *et al.* Clinical evaluation of a new antimetabolite, 6-mercaptopurine, in the treatment of leukemia and allied diseases. Blood 1953; 8:965-99.

[29]   Elion GB. Nobel Lecture in Physiology or Medicine-1988. The purine path to chemotherapy. *In Vitro* Cell Dev Biol 1989; 25:321-30.

[30]   Hitchings GH Jr. Nobel lecture in physiology or medicine--1988. Selective inhibitors of dihydrofolate reductase. *In Vitro* Cell Dev Biol 1989; 25:303-10.

[31]   Clarke DA, Philips FS, Sternberg SS, Stock CC, Elion GB, Hitchings GB. 6-Mercaptopurine: effects in mouse Sarcoma 180 and in normal animals. Cancer Res 1953; 13:593-604.

"Of the agents of limited but definite value in the clinic nearly all were first shown to be active against experimental animal tumors". Dr. C. Chester Stock.

"I maintain that drug-sensitive animal tumor models (when used as 'screens') have uncovered useful anticancer agents that could not have been discovered in any other practical way". Dr. Howard E. Skipper.

CHAPTER 5

The Years of Creativity: 1953-1965. Pre-Clinical

Pierre R. Band[*]

Department of Medicine, McGill University, Montreal, Canada

Abstract: In 1953, the United States National Institutes, including the National Cancer Institute, were assembled in Bethesda. In 1955, a National Cancer Chemotherapy Program was established and scientific panels were formed with the participation of basic and clinical scientists and statisticians. An extensive experimental and clinical drug development program was initiated at the National Cancer Institute. Animal screening models predictive of anticancer drug activity were studied and criteria for pre-clinical toxicology and activity were developed. Important concepts emerged from experimental studies that influenced cancer therapy, including the dose-schedule and first-order kinetics principles, and the effects of anticancer agents on proliferating and resting cells. Under the leadership of Dr. Zubrod, the activities of a triumvirate of clinical scientists, Doctors Frei, Freireich and Holland, initially focussed on the treatment of acute leukemia, following up on Holland's innovative use of a two-drug combination.

Keywords: National Cancer Chemotherapy Program, screening, dose-schedule, first-order kinetics, cell-cycle specific, cell-cycle nonspecific, acute leukemia.

INTRODUCTION

The appreciation that public health was a legitimate concern of government led to the establishment of the National Institutes of Health during the presidency of Franklin D. Roosevelt in the 1930s. Geographically dispersed Institutes of Heart Disease, Arthritis, Cancer, Mental Health, Dentistry and others were assembled in a single specific campus in Bethesda, Maryland, near Washington, D.C. A huge

*Address correspondence to Pierre R. Band: Faculty of Medicine, McGill University, Montreal, Quebec H3G 1Y6, Canada; E-mail: pierre.band@gmail.com

research hospital, the Clinical Center, opened in July 1953. Acute leukemia was an initial focus of clinical research because its outcome was so tragic, some temporary benefits had been seen and cancer cells could be easily and repeatedly sampled.

In 1955, the U.S. Congress gave approval for a National Cancer Chemotherapy Program. This was followed by the foundation at the National Cancer Institute of the Cancer Chemotherapy National Service Center, which provided coordination and administration for the program that "set out on one of the most extensive research programs the world has ever seen [1]". An extensive, integrated drug development program ranging from drug synthesis, screening and pre-clinical investigation to a clinical program initially aimed at testing new anticancer compounds was initiated [2-4]. The experimental and clinical programs were characterized by unique cross-fertilization: findings originating from animal experimentation were tested in the clinic, while clinical questions were investigated experimentally. Five scientific panels — chemistry, screening, pharmacology-biochemistry, clinical studies and endocrinology — were formed with the participation of a wide array of scientists, clinicians and statisticians. Because the pharmaceutical industry plays such an important role in drug development, an industry subcommittee was also set up and a policy was established to protect confidentiality and the proprietary rights of the pharmaceutical companies [4, 5]. That initiative led to a close collaboration between the Cancer Chemotherapy National Service Center and the pharmaceutical industry; over time, a large proportion of the compounds supplied to the screening program originated from pharmaceutical firms. New agents with antitumor activity in animal screening systems were evaluated in a spectrum of human cancer, and cooperative oncology groups were formed. Within three years of its inception, the National Cancer Chemotherapy Program became "without precedent in size, scope, and complexity [3]".

And now it's time to meet the main protagonists of these years of creativity, largely *via* information obtained in 2010 during the author's interviews with Doctors Emil Frei III, Emil J. Freireich and James F. Holland who, at that time, were in their eighties. Regrettably, some of the other pioneers had already died: Doctors Joseph Burchenal, Sidney Farber, David Karnofsky, Frank Schabel Jr., Howard Skipper and Gordon Zubrod.

THE GUIDE

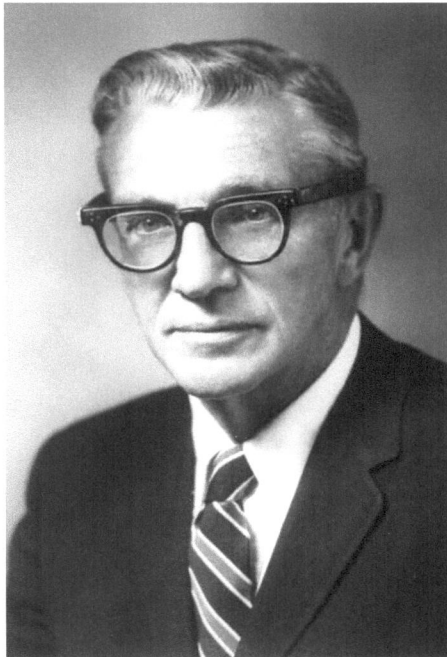

Figure 5.1: Dr. Gordon Zubrod. Photo kindly provided to the author by Dr. Emil J. Freireich.

We've already met Dr. Charles Gordon Zubrod (1914-1999), one of the antimalarial research group members during World War II. Zubrod's background had been in infectious diseases. After the war, he joined the Department of Pharmacology and Experimental Therapeutics at Johns Hopkins University Medical School in Baltimore, Maryland. The department was headed by Dr. Eli K. Marshall (1889-1966), a renowned pharmacologist who had also been a member of the antimalarial research group. At Johns Hopkins University, Zubrod acquired further expertise in the principles of modern pharmacology, issues of translating the information derived from animal experimentation to humans, and the design of clinical trials. After a short period as Director of Clinical Research at the Saint Louis University School of Medicine in Missouri, Zubrod (Fig. **5.1**) became Clinical Director of the National Cancer Institute in 1954. In 1962 he formed the Acute Leukemia Task Force to "engineer the cure of acute leukemia [6]". That initiative, reminiscent of the malaria effort in tackling a single disease and involving the best minds, led to new developments and conceptual advances in cancer chemotherapy. Doctors Burchenal, Farber, Frei, Holland and Skipper were among the initial members of the Task Force [7].

Holland said: "Zubrod was a master of clinical investigation who brought to the National Cancer Institute the concept of the controlled clinical trial. Fundamentally a clinical pharmacologist, he wanted to ensure that we would use drugs correctly. He had cut his teeth on the view that you can have a major program with a goal, and have a highly talented group of people work at all levels of chemical synthesis, pharmacologic assessment and implementation successfully [8]". Frei, who had been Zubrod's Chief Resident at Saint Louis University, told: "He exerted a powerful influence on experimental design, randomized controlled trials and biostatistics [9]", and had written: "Gordon brought a can-be-done attitude to cancer chemotherapy, an attitude not shared by many in the research hierarchy, who believed that the scientific knowledge of cancer generally, and also of developmental pharmacology, was insufficiently developed in 1955 to warrant a large-scale clinical and laboratory program. But Gordon never wavered. From the beginning, it was his vision, his courage, his scientific acumen, and his gentle but firm perseverance that prevailed [10]". Freireich mentioned: "Zubrod was a gentleman, courteous and meticulous; everyone who knew him admired him. He brought from the malaria program the concept of systematically doing chemotherapy: screening in animal models, doing pharmacokinetics, going to early clinical trial in man, developing objective quantitative criteria. He was responsible for all the major advances in the cooperative oncology groups. It was his conception. He had the capacity to recognize good ideas and supported them. He made everything possible. He was a great leader [11]".

THE EXPERIMENTALISTS

The experimentalists played a major role in the development of oncology. Experimental animal models were crucial for testing and for introducing new and effective anticancer drugs in the clinic; important concepts emerged from experimental studies that considerably influenced cancer therapy.

Dr. Lloyd W. Law's (1910-2002) research on drug resistance and combination chemotherapy had a major impact on the design of early clinical studies. Law (Fig. **5.2**, left) also achieved recognition by developing the L1210 mouse leukemia system (the L stands for Law) that became a principal model for predicting drug activity in human acute leukemia and was used extensively in experimental studies aimed at discovering principles of cancer chemotherapy.

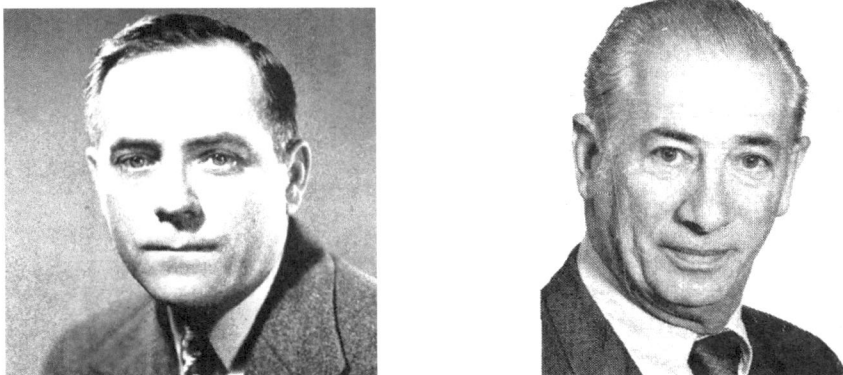

Figure 5.2: Left: Dr. Lloyd Law; photograph taken *circa* 1969; right: Dr. Abraham Goldin; photograph taken *circa* 1979. Courtesy of the National Institutes of Health, United States.

Dr. Abraham Goldin (1911-1988), (Fig. **5.2**, right), a pioneer in experimental chemotherapy, spent his entire career at the National Cancer Institute. Holland said: "He was very devoted to conceptual ways to make drugs behave better. He always thought of drugs, dose, and schedule with characteristics that could easily be translated to man. He was a wonderful feeder of ideas [8]".

Doctors Howard E. Skipper (1915-2006) and Frank M. Schabel Jr. (1918-1983) were a team. As with Doctors Burchenal and Karnofsky, one can't in all justice speak individually of Skipper (Fig. **5.3**, left) and Schabel (Fig **5.3**, right): the two scientists worked at the same institution, the Southern Research Institute in Birmingham, Alabama, and co-authored a number of seminal publications on experimental studies that had a profound impact on cancer medicine.

Holland told: "Skipper was an extraordinary influential man. Schabel did all the experiments, Skipper analyzed the data. At the 13th International Congress of Chemotherapy meeting that took place in Vienna, Austria, in 1983, Schabel was sitting next to me before his talk and told me: 'Jim, when you retire, leave a dog in your office, because after a year he is the only one who will know you', and then a few minutes later he collapsed and died suddenly [8]". Freireich said: "Skipper was like Zubrod, a great leader, open-minded, a great conceptualist; Schabel was the innovator and earthy, he did all the work; every time we had a question, two weeks later we had the answer. We worked very closely with Skipper and Schabel from day one. Schabel died at a meeting I was chairing [11]".

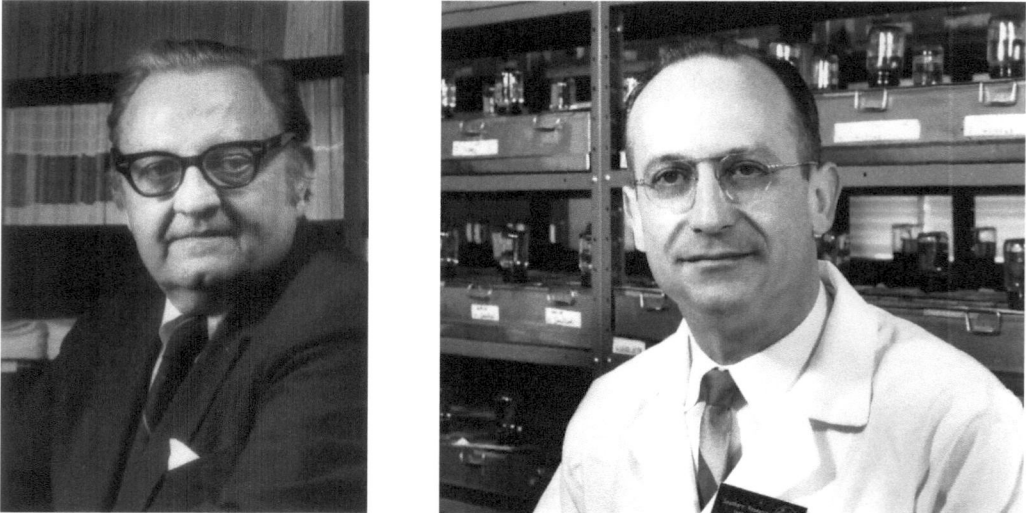

Figure 5.3: Left: Dr. Howard E. Skipper. Right: Dr. Frank M. Schabel Jr. Courtesy of the Southern Research Institute.

"The circumstances surrounding this tragic situation were so extraordinary that the people who were present were motivated to produce a supplementary volume to the journal *Cancer* as a memorial to this event [12]". This volume contains a very moving testimony of Zubrod: "He frequently wrote little notes to me with a reprint or two, apologizing if it was one of his and always saying, 'Gordon-No need to answer'. But I always did. When we returned from vacation, on my desk was one last reprint with its little note that I could not answer [13]".

Dr. Robert W. Bruce (Fig 5.4) graduated in radiation physics before completing a medical degree at the University of Chicago, Illinois, and in 1959 joined the Ontario Cancer Institute and the Department of Medical Biophysics at the University of Toronto in Ontario. He developed a quantitative assay for transplanted lymphoma cells that was designed to measure their sensitivity to radiation in parallel to that of hematopoietic colony-forming units (hematopoietic stem cells).

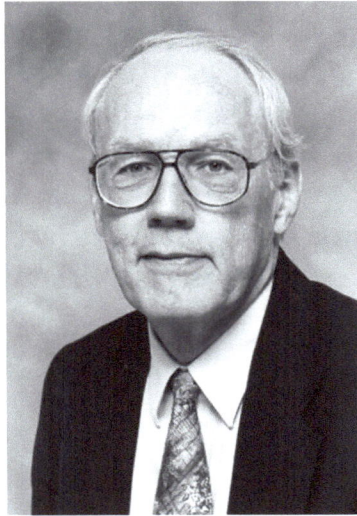

Figure 5.4: Dr. Robert W. Bruce. Photo kindly provided to the author by Dr. Bruce.

A TRIUMVIRATE OF CLINICAL PIONEERS: DOCTORS EMIL FREI III, EMIL J. FREIREICH AND JAMES F. HOLLAND (Fig. 5.5)

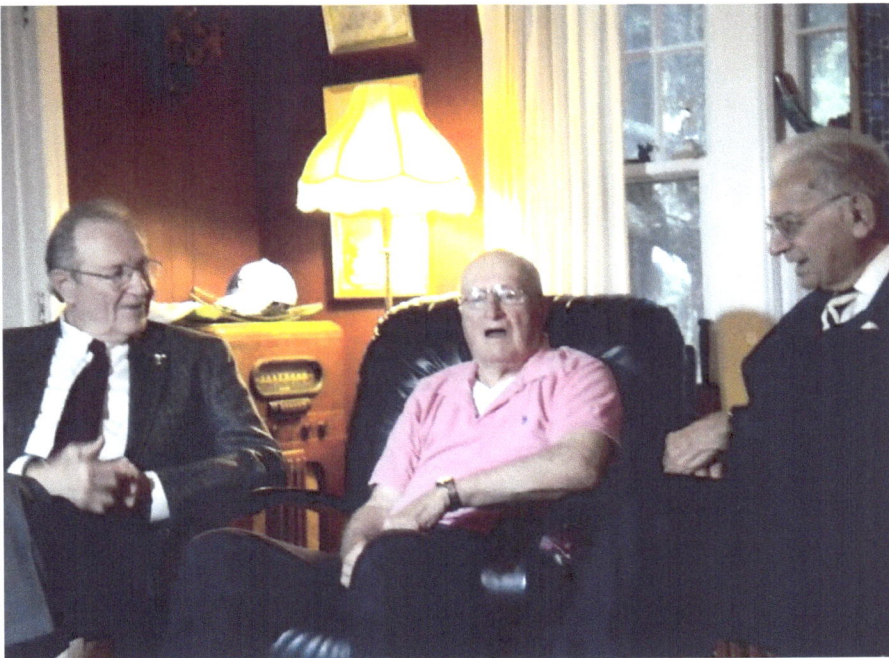

Figure 5.5: From left to right: Doctors Emil J. Freireich, Emil Frei III, James F. Holland. Photo taken by the author; November 2010.

Holland's father was a judge. At Princeton University in New Jersey, Holland studied subjects related to law and biology. He had a wonderful biology teacher who sparked his imagination and so he decided to dedicate himself to medicine rather than law. Holland graduated in medicine at Columbia University's College of Physicians and Surgeons in New York City, where his teacher and mentor was Dr. Alfred Gellhorn (1914-2008), one of the first internists who contributed to research and teaching in cancer medicine. During his residency in internal medicine at Presbyterian Hospital in New York City, Holland read Farber's paper on the treatment of childhood acute lymphocytic leukemia with aminopterin and found it fascinating. After his Army duties, Holland became Chief Resident under Gellhorn, who had become Director of Medical Services at the newly created Francis Delafield Hospital in New York City. There, Holland treated a four-year-old girl who was suffering from acute lymphocytic leukemia with aminopterin and induced her into remission.

At Gellhorn's suggestion, Holland joined the National Cancer Institute. He arrived on July 1, 1953, and was present at the dedication speech of the Clinical Center at the National Institutes of Health. Shortly afterwards, Law, who was a PhD, not a physician, was scheduled to give a scientific seminar to the Scientific Directors about his recent activities in combination chemotherapy. Holland was asked by the Clinical Director of the National Cancer Institute to help Law with the clinical aspects of his presentation. That was the first time the two met and they became close friends. Law had used a purine analogue, 8-azaguanine, combined with aminopterin, showing that the combination prolonged the survival of mice with lymphocytic leukemia longer than the two drugs given sequentially. Holland set up the first combination chemotherapy of acute leukemia using methotrexate, which Goldin had shown to have a better therapeutic index than aminopterin, and 6-mercaptopurine, a different purine analogue that was better tolerated than 8-azaguanine. According to Holland, "based on the simplified rationale of the time, if one-third of the patients responded to methotrexate and one-third responded to 6-mercaptopurine, then 1 in 9 patients should respond to both and potentially get cured. I treated the daughter of the Chaplain of the U.S. Senate and she did particularly well [8]". While at the National Cancer Institute, Holland used this combination for the treatment of several patients with acute leukemia.

Emil Frei III comes from a family of artists who founded a well-known stained glass company in Saint Louis. "I was first enamoured by sports and played on the St-Mary's High School football and baseball teams in South Saint Louis. One of my teachers took an interest in me and imparted in me his knowledge and enthusiasm for medicine and mathematics [9]". Frei graduated in medicine from Yale University in New Haven, Connecticut, and went on to postgraduate studies in medicine and pathology at Saint Louis University. As Chief-Resident, Frei was tutored by a newly appointed associate professor with an interest in pharmacology, infectious diseases and clinical trials: Dr. Charles Gordon Zubrod, who became his mentor. When Zubrod came to the National Cancer Institute, he invited Frei to join him. In 1955, Frei arrived at the National Cancer Institute where he became Chief of the Leukemia Section and subsequently Chief of Medicine.

Nothing can surpass the views of this physician, to whom all medical oncologists are indebted, than those of the colleagues who shared with him the historical development of the field. Holland said of Frei:

> Tom is an extraordinary intelligent man, exceptionally good at organization, exceptionally good at seeing things strategically. I gave the dedicatory speech when his bust was unveiled at the Dana Farber Cancer Institute in Boston, Massachusetts. I said that he had rainbow vision; that when other people saw things in black and white, Tom could see them in color; everything was really elaborately alive from his point of view. And he could see over barriers much better than others could. The average person puts enough rocks on the pile to see over the barrier and what do they see: another barrier farther along. But Tom could see over a barrier and deduce where the eventual road would lie. He probably has trained more academic medical oncologists than anybody. And essentially all his trainees went on in academic life. He has been a passionate advocate of combination chemotherapy. Tom is a distinguished medical oncologist from a point of view of knowledge, of being able to synthesize things, to instil and inculcate in people a desire to work hard, but he also possesses a tremendous ability to see ahead and to act strategically. He is easy to work with. I have worked with him for 50 years. He always listens. He is

honest, never a blemish, never the slightest deviation from open communication; an admirable man [8].

And Freireich added: "Tom Frei has an extraordinary ability to recognize things that make changes in the way we think. It takes open-minded intelligence to be adaptable to new ideas; Tom Frei has that characteristic. Nothing that I did would have ever been done had it not been for Tom Frei and Gordon Zubrod [11]".

You may be wondering why Frei was known as Tom rather than Emil. Freireich explained: "His father, Emil Frei Jr., and his grandfather, Emil Frei, were both alive when Emil Frei III was young. So when he was called, one did not know who was being addressed. The family arbitrarily called him 'Tom' after Tom Sawyer, both children of the Mississippi river [11]".

Emil Freireich was two years old in 1929, when his father died suddenly and the Wall Street crash occurred. Freireich, a born storyteller, relates the story himself, but unfortunately we can't hear the intonations:

> I grew-up on the streets with the other kids in that Chicago Ghetto where everybody was poor and starving. At the age of 10, I developed tonsillitis and was attended by a physician who came to our ghetto-type apartment, reassured me and prescribed . . . ice cream! He was wearing a suit and a tie. In my young life, I never saw a man with a suit and a tie and from that day forward, I dreamt of becoming a famous doctor. In school, my major was typing and shorthand because my mother thought that with these subjects I could get a job as a secretary. During my senior year, a PhD in physics came deliberately in the ghetto high school to teach physics to kids in trouble and save them. That was his mission in life. We had a physics contest and I won it. This teacher then called me to his office: "Freireich, I think you should go to college. I will write you a letter. If you get 25 dollars, you will go to university and I will tell you how to do it". A lady who used money to do good things in the ghetto gave my mother 25 dollars and this is how I attended college. In those years, several pre-medical students failed the course that determined whether you'd go to medicine or not. This course was physics, which

turned out to be my forte. I was accepted in medical school and then went to Cook County Hospital in Chicago. Medicine was an eye-opener for me. It was so complicated; I was overwhelmed by the knowledge required. I took a residency in medicine at Rush Presbyterian Hospital and became Chief Resident. One day the Head of Medicine asked what I wanted to do. I want to be a family doctor. "Well," he said, "you had very good recommendations from all attending physicians, what in medicine are you less familiar with?" "Well," I said, "I don't want to offend you, but the professor who taught us hematology is a jerk, so I know nothing about hematology". He replied: "No problem, you have to go to Boston and learn all the new scientific knowledge in hematology", which I did. In 1955, there was a doctor draft because the military was short of doctors, and I became a second lieutenant in the inactive army reserve! About a week later, the Dean of our Medical School, Dr. Chester S. Keefer (1897-1972) called me to his office. He told me that he was the United States Under-Secretary for Health and asked if I had heard of the National Institutes of Health. No, Sir. "Well," he said, "there is this place near Washington where they just built a new hospital called the Clinical Center, it is pretty much empty and my job is to populate it with brilliant young physician scientists, and I am told that you are doing a very good job. I want you to go to Washington and meet a few people". The next day I met Gordon Zubrod who inquired about my specialty. I am a hematologist. Zubrod thought a little, scratched his head and said: "Freireich what you ought to do is to cure leukemia". Yes Sir, I said, after all I was in the Army! When I arrived at the National Cancer Institute in 1955, Zubrod told me that I had an office on the 12th floor. So I went up to the 12th floor, walked down the corridor and saw a sign: Emil Frei. Damn, I thought, isn't this like the Government, they can't even spell my name! I opened the door and here was this tall skinny guy with no hair. I said "you took my office". And Frei replied: "Your office is next door". And there we were bound together [11].

Indeed they were, and not only by the similarity of their names. As Frei used to say, "Freireich is perfect in all ways save that his name is overly long [14]". In an eloquent tribute, Frei wrote: "The real meaning of friendship, of collegiality, of working towards a common goal, of sharing failure, and of experiencing the exhilaration of high achievement defies analysis. On a personal level, Freireich's collegiality has been to me, invaluable, and the many moments in discussion, of insights, of learning together, and of laughing together were precious [14].

SCREENING

In Chapter 4, we saw the importance of screening for the discovery of compounds with anticancer activity. Screening became a major part of the drug development program of the Cancer Chemotherapy National Service Center "probably the largest drug screening program in the history of medicine [3]". The main goal was to develop experimental animal models predictive of activity against human cancer.

The first recorded attempt to transplant a tumor dates back to 1773 when a French surgeon, Dr. Bernard Peyrilhe (1737-1804), transplanted about 6 grams of breast cancer tissue under the skin of a dog. Judging from Peyrilhe's description, a severe infection ensued: "the poor creature was perpetually howling; at length my maid, disgusted by the stench of the ulcer, and softened by the cries of the animal, put an end to his life, and thus prevented my observing the ultimate effects of this disease [15]". A century passed before a Russian veterinarian, Mstislav A. Novinsky (1841-1914), performed the first successful transplant of a malignant tumor from a dog into a puppy in 1876 [16]. Subsequently, tumor transplantation was successfully performed in rodents by Arthur Hanau (1858-1900) in Switzerland, Henri Moreau (1860-date of death unknown) in France, and Leo Loeb (1869-1959) in the United States [17, 18]. However, Carl O. Jensen (1877-1953), a Danish veterinary surgeon, is credited with spearheading the systematic experimental transplantation of tumors with animals of the same species [19] that marked "the beginning of experimental cancer research [20]" which, together with the development of inbred strains of animals [21], made experimental animal models for drug screening and evaluation possible.

In 1955, the screening systems used to predict for antitumor activity were reviewed in a publication known as the Gellhorn-Hirschberg report, which collated the analysis of 27 compounds across 74 screening systems [22]. No system had better predictive value for human activity of the compounds then known than transplanted tumors in mice. Based on the report, the Cancer Chemotherapy National Service Center initially selected a spectrum of 3 animal tumor systems (Leukemia L1210, Sarcoma 180 and Mammary adenocarcinoma 755) as a primary screen for drug activity, and developed specifications for screening antitumor compounds [23]. The predictive value of screening systems is dependent on correlation with clinical activity. While it was soon realized that the leukemia L1210 model selected for most chemotherapeutic drugs active against acute leukemia in humans [24], correlation with most cancers would have to await the findings of clinical trials. Screening systems were periodically re-evaluated as clinical data became available to validate the information derived from animal models, and as the characteristics of tumor growth were being unravelled [25-28]. A major review of the cancer chemotherapy screening program also occurred under the auspices of the Acute Leukemia Task Force [25]. As a result, animal screening systems were modified, with some eliminated and newer ones added. For instance, leukemia L1210 remained the model of choice for initial screening, Sarcoma 180 and Mammary adenocarcinoma 755 were replaced by other tumor systems, and the leukemia P388 mouse model was added to screen natural products [25, 28].

CRITERIA FOR DRUG TOXICITY AND THERAPEUTIC ACTIVITY

Drugs that are active against cancer also produce toxic effects on the host. Experimental animal systems designed to select anticancer agents active against human cancer therefore require quantitative measures of both toxicity and therapeutic effects, with additional quantitative information on the relative safety of the compound. Objective endpoints for toxicity and therapeutic effects were developed for both leukemia and solid tumor animal models [29, 30]. The main toxicity endpoint characterized was the maximum tolerated dose defined as the lethal dose 10, the dose that kills 10% of the treated animals. The minimum effective dose or therapeutic endpoint was considered, for leukemia, to be the dose producing a 40% increase in the life span of treated animals compared to untreated controls. For solid tumors, the minimum effective dose consisted of a 90% tumor inhibition, which is the ratio of tumor weight or volume between treated and control animals equal to 10%. The therapeutic index, the ratio of a maximum tolerated dose to a minimum effective dose, was also taken into consideration. Its importance lies in the fact that it reflects the relative safety of a drug: the higher the ratio, the greater the margin of safety. For example, if the maximum tolerated dose is 1 mg and the minimum effective dose is 0.5 mg, a ratio of 2, the therapeutic effect occurs at half the maximum tolerated dose; in the case of a minimum effective dose of 1.0 mg, the therapeutic effect would occur at the maximum tolerated dose. Most agents of clinical value were found to have a therapeutic index of 2 or greater [5].

Once a drug passed the screening tests successfully, it would undergo pre-clinical toxicologic and pharmacologic evaluation [30]. It is interesting to note that the toxicity and therapeutic criteria established were fairly stringent, as may be inferred from the fact that only 2 of about 1000 synthetic compounds screened proceeded to pharmacologic assessment [31]. As part of the Acute Leukemia Task Force program, a Pharmacology Subcommittee was set up to establish guidelines and criteria for conducting pharmacologic studies of chemotherapeutic drugs [32].

PRINCIPLES OF CHEMOTHERAPY OF CLINICAL RELEVANCE DERIVED FROM EXPERIMENTAL STUDIES

1. Drug Resistance and Combination Chemotherapy

Drug resistance is one of the major limitations of the therapeutic effect of anticancer agents. This problem was commented upon in the initial report of complete remissions induced by a chemotherapeutic drug in a human malignancy [33]. The development of resistance to anticancer drugs was subsequently described in experimental leukemia of mice [34, 35] and in other tumor systems [36]. In studies using the L1210 leukemia model, Law showed that malignant cells developed drug resistance by spontaneous mutations and selection [36, 37]. Spontaneous mutations arose independently of the presence of the drug, whereas the drug selected the resistant variant by eradicating the sensitive cells, leaving the resistant ones behind to proliferate.

Combination chemotherapy was pioneered in studies by Law and Goldin in the early 1950s [38, 39]. The reasoning went that cells that were spontaneously resistant to two chemotherapeutic drugs would have a very low probability of occurrence; thus, in order to minimize resistance, two or more drugs that acted independently on different targets and given simultaneously should have a therapeutic effect superior to either drug used alone. At the time, the rationale for combination chemotherapy was based on biochemical considerations, mainly on the blockade of metabolic pathways leading to constituents essential to cell growth [40, 41].

2. A Recurrent Theme: How to Achieve Selective Toxicity of Chemotherapeutic Drugs for Malignant Cells

Dose-Schedule

In a seminal study designed to ascertain the effect of chemotherapy at different stages of the disease, Goldin *et al.* inoculated mice with L1210 leukemia cells. Treatment with methotrexate was then initiated at an earlier (day 5) and more advanced (day 9) stage. In early disease, it was observed that the optimal administration of methotrexate was every four days. At that schedule of drug administration, a higher dose was tolerated leading to a greater increase in life span compared to the drug given daily [42]. At day 9, however, when the leukemic cell population was greater and the mouse was clearly sicker, daily treatment was superior. As was aptly emphasized, the therapeutic property of an anticancer agent is not fixed but "may be altered by the manner in which the drug is employed [43]". The dose-schedule concept would have a lasting influence on clinical cancer chemotherapy.

First-Order Kinetics

In 1937, Furth and Kahn showed that the inoculation of one leukemia cell could lead to cell proliferation and death from leukemia in recipient mice [44]. This observation was overlooked, however, possibly because the publication occurred at a time when therapy was limited to potassium arsenite (Fowler's solution), which had been used since the 19th century with some activity against leukemia [45]. In the more propitious era of the Acute Leukemia Task Force, Skipper and colleagues not only repeated and confirmed Furth and Kahn's observation, but also deduced from it therapeutic principles destined to have a major impact on clinical cancer chemotherapy. If indeed one leukemia cell can be lethal, then all leukemic cells must be eradicated if cure is to be the aim. Consequently, quantitative data must be acquired on the kinetics of leukemia cell proliferation and the cell-kill effect of chemotherapy. This was achieved using the L1210 leukemia model in studies reported in two major publications [46, 47]. First a logarithmically increasing number of leukemia cells were inoculated into mice: 1, 10, 100 and so on up to 1,000,000. It was observed that: 1) After an initial lag time, the growth rate of leukemia cells was exponential for all levels of cells injected, with a cell doubling time of about half-a-day; 2) The number of days between the time of inoculation and death was inversely proportional to the number of cells injected, 1.8 days on average between two consecutive log-dose levels. With this information at hand, treatment was initiated using a single fixed dose for a given chemotherapeutic agent. It was found that the cell-kill effect was constant, whatever the number of leukemia cells present at the time treatment was started; for instance, for a therapeutic effect of 90%, if treatment was initiated when the cell burden was 1,000,000, the same 90% cell-kill effect was found when treatment was initiated when the cell burden was 100,000; 3) The percentage of cell-kill varied directly with the dose, being highest at the maximum tolerated dose; at maximum tolerated dose, single doses administered intermittently gave superior results compared to daily doses. The constant percentage cell-kill of a given dose of a given chemotherapeutic drug was referred to as a first-order kinetic reaction from its similarity with other natural phenomena [48].

The main clinical corollaries of these observations were that to cure a malignant disease: 1) All malignant cells must be killed, barring the possibility of eradication of a small number of residual cells by host immune reaction; 2) Treatment must be initiated at the earliest time possible when the number of malignant cells is lower; 3) Intermittent high-dose chemotherapy should be used instead of smaller daily doses to induce a higher fractional cell-kill.

Skipper's papers, as noted above, have been widely quoted in the scientific literature. Less well known, is a publication that reflected his sense of humor. He came up with the "Peck-Order of Scientific Status", how the scientific community ranks the social status of researchers on a scale of 1 to 10, 1 being the highest. According to this ranking, status is inversely related to the size of the object under study. On the lowest end of the scale is the clinician whose object of study is the human being; in the middle is the biochemist whose concern is with large molecules; the nuclear physicist involved with atomic particles ranks second; way on top we find the theoretical mathematician whose object of study is weightless [49].

Cell-Cycle Effects

Bruce and colleagues at the Ontario Cancer Institute (now Cancer Care Ontario) in Toronto investigated the effects of chemotherapeutic drugs using the spleen-colony assay, an ingenious technique that makes it possible to simultaneous study a drug on the proliferative capacity of normal and malignant cells. The authors compared the effectiveness of various chemotherapeutic agents against normal bone marrow cells, both proliferating and resting, with clonogenic lymphoma cells, the proliferating fraction of the latter being higher. Three patterns of responses were noted (Fig. **5.6**).

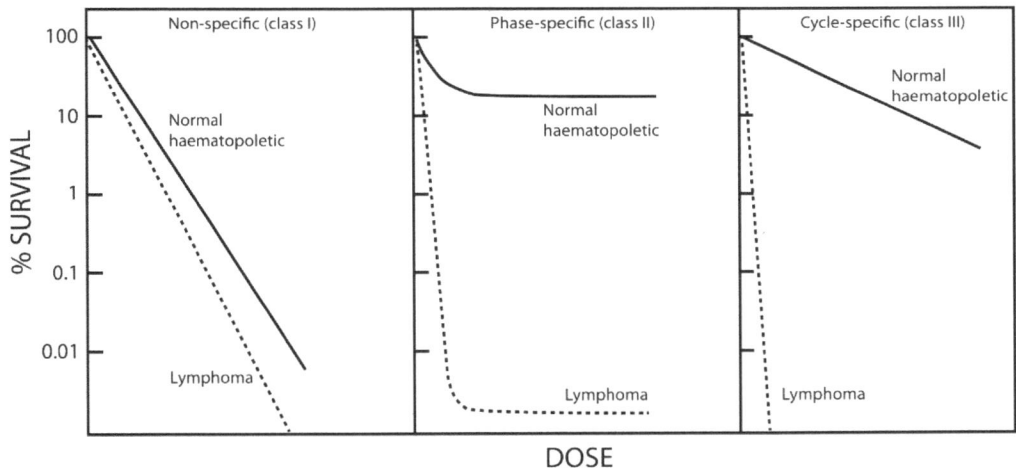

Figure 5.6: Patterns of response to chemotherapeutic agents (see text); Fig. **1** in: Hill BT, Baserga R. The cell cycle and its signifcance for cancer treatment. Cancer Treat Rev 1975; 2, 159-75; reference 52. Reproduced with permission from Elsevier.

Class I drugs showed an exponential dose-related cell-kill that was similar for normal and lymphoma cells. Class II agents induced a dose-related decrease in cell survival down to a constant value beyond which no further inhibition occurred despite increasing doses. The constant values differed markedly, however, being much lower for malignant cells. Class III drugs showed an exponential cell-kill for both types of cells, but steeper for lymphoma cells. The following interpretation for these distinctive patterns was offered. Class I drugs, which must be equally toxic for proliferating and resting cells, were referred to as cell-cycle nonspecific. Since Class II drugs only kill cells in one phase of the cell cycle, those not entering this phase during drug exposure were unaffected; agents of this class were called cell-cycle phase-specific. Class III drugs kill cells in both the proliferating and resting phases, but are more toxic for proliferating cells; thus, cell-kill is directly related to the proliferative fraction; this class of agents was described as cell-cycle specific. [50].

As was pointed out: "These experimental findings demonstrate the cellular basis for the selective toxicity of high-dose intermittent chemotherapy for malignant cells and suggest that . . . phase-specific and cycle-specific agents should be administered in short, intensive courses, using maximal tolerated dose [51]". Bruce's study also provided a rationale for drug selection with respect to tumor growth rates and for combination chemotherapy. The cell-kinetics effects of chemotherapeutic agents were subsequently updated with details on their site of action relative to the different phases the cell cycle [52].

Protecting Against Host Lethal Toxicity While Improving Therapeutic Index

The anticancer activity of methotrexate, like that of many other chemotherapeutic agents, is limited by bone marrow toxicity. Burchenal reported that folic acid and leucovorin (citrovorum factor), a reduced derivative of folic acid beyond the chemical step that is inhibited by folic antagonists, prevented the chemotherapeutic effects of methotrexate on mouse leukemia [53, 54]. Using the L1210 mouse leukemia model, Goldin subsequently showed that delayed administration of leucovorin 12 hours after methotrexate protected against the lethal toxicity of the drug without affecting its therapeutic activity [55]. Higher doses of methotrexate could thus be given, with improved survival of the treated animals.

REFERENCES

[1]   MacGregor AB. The search for a chemical cure for cancer. Med Hist 1966; 10:374-85.
[2]   Endicott KM. The chemotherapy program. J Natl Cancer Inst 1957; 19:275-93.

[3]   Endicott KM. The national cancer chemotherapy program. J Chronic Dis 1958; 8:171-7.

[4]   Zubrod CG, Schepartz S, Leiter J, Endicott KM, Carrese LM, Baker CG. The chemotherapy program of the National Cancer Institute: history, analysis and plans. Cancer Chemother Rep 1966; 50:349-540.

[5]   Wood HB Jr. Selection of agents for the tumor screen. Cancer Chemother Rep 1971; Part 3; 2:9-22.

[6]   Zubrod CG. Origins and development of chemotherapy research at the National Cancer Institute. Cancer Treat Rep 1984; 68:9-19.

[7]   Zubrod CG. Combinations of drugs in the treatment of acute leukemias. Proc R Soc Med 1965; 58 (11 Part 2):988-90.

[8]   Author's interview with Dr. James F. Holland.

[9]   Author's interview with Dr. Emil Frei III.

[10]   Emil Frei III. In memoriam. C. Gordon Zubrod, MD. J Clin Oncol 1999; 17:1331-33.

[11]   Author's interview with Dr. Emil J. Freireich.

[12]   Freireich EJ. A memorial issue for Dr. Frank M. Schabel Jr. Introduction. Cancer 1984; 54 (Suppl 1):1132-3.

[13]   Zubrod CG. Testimonials. Ibid p. 1147.

[14]   Frei E 3rd. Confrontation, passion, and personalization. Emil J. Freireich. Clin Cancer Res 1997; 3:2554-62.

[15]   A dissertation on cancerous disease by B. Peyrilhe. Translated from Latin with notes. London: J. Wilkie 1777; pp. 45-46.

[16]   Shabad LM, Ponomarkov VI. Mstislav Novinsky, pioneer of tumour transplantation. Cancer Lett 1976; 2:1-3.

[17]   Schoenberg BS, Schoenberg DG. Of mice and men, of triumph and tragedy, of murine models of malignant disease. Surg Gynecol Obstet 1975; 141:933-7.

[18]   Heller JR. Cancer chemotherapy, history and present status. Bull NY Acad Med 1962; 38:348-63.

[19]   Anonymous. Obituary. Carl Olaf Jensen, MD. Br Med J 1934; 2:535.

[20]   Foulds L. Neoplastic development. Volume 1. London: Academic Press 1969; pp. 7-14.

[21]   Griswold, DP Jr, Harrison SD Jr. Tumor models in drug development. Cancer Metastasis Rev 1991; 10:255-261.

[22]   Gellhorn A, Hirschberg E. Investigation of diverse systems for cancer chemotherapy screening. Cancer Res 1955; 3 (Suppl 1) 3:1-125.

[23]   Cancer Chemotherapy National Service Center. Specifications for screening chemical agents and natural products against animal tumors. Cancer Chemotherapy Rep 1959; 1:42-64.

[24]   Frei E 3rd. Comparisons of activities of antitumor agents in selected human and rodent tumor systems. Cancer Chemother Rep 1962; 16:19-24.

[25]   Goldin A, Serpick AA, Mantel N. Experimental screening procedures and clinical predictability value. Cancer Chemother Rep 1966; 50:173-218.

[26]   Shepartz SA. Screening. Cancer Chemother Rep 1971 Part 3; 2:3-8.

[27]   Schabel FM Jr. Screening, the cornerstone of chemotherapy. Cancer Chemother Rep1972; 2:309-13.

[28]   Venditti JM. Working session report: *in vivo-in vitro* screening. Cancer Chemother Rep 1972; 3:57-62.

[29] Goldin A, Venditti JM, Mantel N. Pre clinical screening and evaluation of agents for the chemotherapy of cancer: a review. Cancer Res 1961; 21:1334-51.

[30] Skipper HE, Schmidt LH. A manual on quantitative drug evaluation in experimental tumor systems. I. Background, description of criteria, and presentation of quantitative therapeutic data on various classes of drugs obtained in diverse experimental tumor systems. Cancer Chemother Rep 1962; 17:1-143.

[31] The National program of cancer chemotherapy research. Cancer Chemother Rep 1959; 1:5-19.

[32] Oliverio VT. Pharmacology in the chemotherapy drug development program of the National Cancer Institute. Cancer Chemother Rep 1971 Part 3; 2:73-9.

[33] Goodman LS, Wintrobe MM, Dameshek W, Goodman MJ, Gilman A, McLennan MT. Nitrogen mustard therapy; use of methyl-bis (beta-chloroethyl) amine hydrochloride and tris (beta-chloroethyl) amine hydrochloride for Hodgkin's disease, lymphosarcoma, leukemia and certain allied and miscellaneous disorders. JAMA 1946; 132:126-32.

[34] Burchenal JH, Robinson E, Johnston SF, Kushida MN. The induction of resistance to 4-amino-N10-methylpteorylglutamic acid in a strain of transmitted mouse leukemia. Science 1950; 111:116.

[35] Law LW, Boyle PJ. Development of resistance to folic acid antagonists in a transplantable lymphoid leukemia. Proc Soc Exp Biol Med 1950; 74:599-602.

[36] Law LW. Differences between cancers in terms of evolution of drug resistance. Cancer Res 1956; 16:698-716.

[37] Law LW. Origin of the resistance of leukaemic cells to folic acid antagonists. Nature 1952; 169:628-9.

[38] Law LW. Effects of combinations of antileukemic agents on an acute lymphocytic leukemia of mice. Cancer Res 1952; 13:871-8.

[39] Goldin A, Greenspan EM, Schoenbach EB. Studies on the mechanism of action of chemotherapeutic agents in cancer. VI. Synergistic (additive) action of drugs on a transplantable leukemia in mice. Cancer 1952; 5:153-60.

[40] Skipper HE, Heidelberger C, Welch AD. Some biochemical problems of cancer chemotherapy. Nature 1957; 179:1159-62.

[41] Goldin A, Mantel N. The employment of combinations of drugs in the chemotherapy of neoplasia: a review. Cancer Res 1957; 17:635-54.

[42] Goldin A, Humphreys SR, Mantel N, Venditti JM. Modification of treatment of schedules in the management of advanced mouse leukemia with amethopterin. J Natl Cancer Inst 1956; 17:203-12.

[43] Goldin A, Venditti JM, Humphreys SR, Shuster L, Darrow RA, Mantel N. Advanced leukemia as a tool for chemotherapeutic studies. Acta Unio Int Contra Cancrum 1960; 16:642-50.

[44] Furth J, Kahn MC. The transmission of leukemia of mice with a single cell. Am J Cancer 1937; 31:276-82.

[45] Lissauer H. Zwei Fälle von Leucaemie. Berl Klin Wschr 1865; 2:403-4.

[46] Skipper HE, Schabel FM Jr, Wilcox WS. Experimental evalutation of potential anticancer agents. XIII. On the criteria and kinetics associated with "curability" of experimental leukemias. Cancer Chemother Rep 1964; 35:3-111.

[47] Skipper HE, Schabel FM Jr, Wilcox WS. Experimental evaluation of potential anticancer agents. XIV. Further study of certain basic concepts underlying chemotherapy of leukemia. Cancer Chemother Rep 1965; 45:5-28.

[48]   Wilcox WS. The last surviving cancer cell: the chances of killing it. Cancer Chemother Rep 1966; 50:541-2.

[49]   Skipper HE. Philosophy at the preclinical level. Cancer Chemother Rep 1962; 16:587-8.

[50]   Bruce WR, Meeker BE, Valeriote FA. Comparison of the sensitivity of normal hematopoietic and transplanted lymphoma colony-forming cells to chemotherapeutic agents administered *in vivo*. J Natl Cancer Inst 1966; 37:233-45.

[51]   Bergsagel DE. An assessment of massive-dose chemotherapy of malignant disease. CMAJ 1971; 104:31-6.

[52]   Hill BT, Baserga R. The cell cycle and its significance for cancer treatment. Cancer Treat Rev 1975; 2:159-75.

[53]   Burchenal JH, Kushida MN, Johnston SF, Cremer MA. Prevention of chemotherapeutic effects of 4-amino-N10-methyl-pteroylglutamic acid on mouse leukemia by pteroylglutamic acid. Proc Soc Exp Biol Med 1949; 71:559-62.

[54]   Burchenal JH, Babcock GM, Broquist HP, Jukes TH. Prevention of chemotherapeutic effects of 4-amino-N10-methyl-pteroylglutamic acid on mouse leukemia by citrovorum factor. Proc Soc Exp Biol Med 1950; 74:735-7.

[55]   Goldin A, Venditti JM, Kline I, Mantel N. Eradication of leukaemic cells (L1210) by methotrexate and methotrexate plus citrovorum factor. Nature 1966; 212:1548-50.

"For a long time to come many, if not most, aspects of any cancer chemotherapy program will require complicated and ingenious experimental and clinical research, correlation, and interpretation by the best minds available". Dr. Gordon Zubrod.

"Cancer clinical trials moved from a largely qualitative effort to a quantitative science, that is, a science that provided information on which one could build incrementally and quantitatively toward cure". Dr. Emil Frei III.

CHAPTER 6

The Years of Creativity: 1953-1965. Clinical

Pierre R. Band[*]

Department of Medicine, McGill University, Montreal, Canada

Abstract: During the 1950s and early 1960s, several principles of chemotherapy were established, principally from methodical studies in childhood acute lymphocytic leukemia carried out within the setting of cooperative oncology groups. Combination chemotherapy, first initiated at the National Cancer Institute, led to a protocol comparing two drugs *versus* one; the results showed that two drugs given together were better than their sequential administration. The dose-schedule principle and first-order kinetic action of chemotherapeutic drugs were successfully studied in the clinic. A leap forward occurred with the demonstration that the effects of new chemotherapeutic agents could be tested in patients in clinical remission. Imaginative study designs were conceived leading to the identification of different phases of therapy: induction, maintenance and periodic reinduction. A continuous-flow blood cell separator was developed; granulocye and platelet transfusions were used to effectively reduce death from infections and hemorrhages; methods of treating meningeal leukemia became available. With these advances, long-term duration of unmaintained remission was seen in children with acute lymphocytic leukemia. Also, for the first time, the cure of a metastatic solid tumor in human, choriocarcinoma, was achieved.

Keywords: Acute lymphocytic leukemia, combination chemotherapy, induction, maintenance, reinduction, granulocyte and platelet transfusions, meningeal leukemia, choriocarcinoma.

*Address correspondence to Pierre R. Band: Faculty of Medicine, McGill University, Montreal, Quebec H3G 1Y6, Canada; E-mail: pierre.band@gmail.com

THE CLIMATE

Reminiscing on the initial clinical trial of nitrogen mustard, Gilman wrote: "In the minds of most physicians the administration of drugs, other than an analgesic, in the treatment of malignant disease was the act of a charlatan [1]". In the mid-50s, the prevailing attitude of physicians towards their colleagues in medicine involved in the treatment of cancer patients was also one of scepticism if not outright antagonism. A commonly heard remark was: "Why poison patients who are dying anyway?" Frei's spontaneous reply to the question: "What was your main challenge?" attests in the author's mind to the prevailing attitude of the medical establishment at the time and to the negative impact it had: "We always had to face that barrier of pessimism as I called it, which affected our patients, our trainees, our own attitude towards things. So to provide leadership in the cancer area required a lot of courage and foresight and the ability to turn off the pessimism that existed. It is not surprising given that position, that the early medical oncologists were all optimists no matter how difficult the situation was, not a trivial attitude but within the bounds of reality. You had to believe that it could be done. Nothing is more unphilosophical than to say that because it has not been done it cannot be done [2]".

This problem was compounded by the fact that the medical schools of the day offered no teaching in cancer medicine. As Dr. Bayard Clarkson said: "Internists would give wonderful bedside lectures, but when it came to cancer they held their tongue [3]". When asked what teaching he had received on cancer, Freireich exclaimed: "We did not even know the word! [4]".

It is against this background and against all odds that the road to the specialty of medical oncology began.

CHILDHOOD ACUTE LYMPHOCYTIC LEUKEMIA: A PARADIGM FOR CANCER CHEMOTHERAPY

Inspired by Law's pioneering studies of combination chemotherapy in mouse leukemia, Holland designed a protocol combining methotrexate and 6-mercaptopurine for the treatment of patients with acute leukemia. Zubrod arrived at the National Cancer Institute in the fall of 1954, about one month before Holland left to join Roswell Park Memorial Institute. They immediately developed a warm friendship. "'I don't have a program in acute leukemia,' Zubrod told me, 'would you mind if I continued yours?' This magnanimous gesture was the initial seed of collaborative cancer research in the United States and marked the beginning of a path leading to the cure of childhood acute leukemia [5]".

Protocol 1

In 1955, Holland, Zubrod, and Frei, who by then had arrived at the National Cancer Institute, began to discuss a new protocol for acute leukemia. Zubrod indicated that a one-arm study would not advance knowledge, and that the combination of methotrexate and 6-mercaptopurine should be tested against methotrexate to investigate the potential superiority of combination chemotherapy. Holland argued that it would be unethical not to go with the best treatment available. A compromise was reached with the suggestion that Goldin's intermittent high dosing of methotrexate *versus* daily methotrexate, both combined with 6-mercaptopurine, might make a difference. As part of the program in acute leukemia, Holland, Frei and Burchenal on behalf of the Clinical Studies Panel of the Cancer Chemotherapy National Service Center, established objective criteria for complete and partial remission and for disease progression. These objective quantitative criteria for evaluating response were first presented at the Sixth International Hematology Congress and later published under the name of the Clinical Studies Panel executive secretary [6]. Finally, a protocol, Protocol 1 [7], was written by Dr. Richard T. Silver, at the time a clinical associate at the National Cancer Institute, because he was the only one who knew how to type! The protocol, which involved clinicians and statisticians, was designed according to the principles of clinical trials pioneered in Great Britain [8-10]; it included, among others, random individual patient allocation to treatment groups and objective criteria for response evaluation. Two regimens were compared: 6-mercaptopurine daily with methotrexate 2.5 mg given daily *versus* 6-mercaptopurine daily with methotrexate 7.5 mg administered every three days. Both children and adults with acute lymphocytic and acute myelocytic leukemias were included. We should remind ourselves, as Freireich noted, "leukemia was just leukemia; we did not know the differences between the natural history of acute leukemia in adults and children [4]". The results showed no significant difference between the treatment groups, though patients receiving both drugs given daily survived a bit longer.

It must have been disappointing not to confirm Goldin's dose-schedule principle in the clinic, but with the help of hindsight, only the methotrexate schedule was truly modified, the total doses of the drug being the same in both groups. Two important observations were made, however. First, responses differed according to the morphologic type of leukemia, with all responses in children occurring in those with acute lymphocytic leukemia. Secondly, survival duration was directly related to the time spent in remission. Protocol 1, in which three different institutions participated (Fig. **6.1**), was the first ever organized cancer cooperative multi-institutional clinical trial; it not only investigated combination chemotherapy but also set the stage for the creation of cooperative oncology groups. On the other hand, it had what could be qualified as growing pains, drawbacks that were subsequently corrected. Specifically, about one-quarter of the patients entered in the study were excluded due to protocol violation, and of those treated according to protocol, close to one-quarter had received prior treatment with the drugs under study.

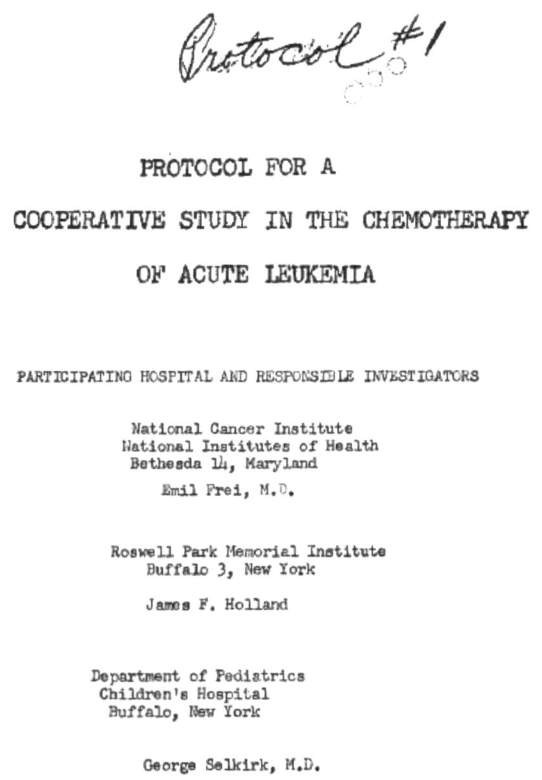

Protocol #1

PROTOCOL FOR A

COOPERATIVE STUDY IN THE CHEMOTHERAPY

OF ACUTE LEUKEMIA

PARTICIPATING HOSPITAL AND RESPONSIBLE INVESTIGATORS

National Cancer Institute
National Institutes of Health
Bethesda 14, Maryland

Emil Frei, M.D.

Roswell Park Memorial Institute
Buffalo 3, New York

James F. Holland

Department of Pediatrics
Children's Hospital
Buffalo, New York

George Selkirk, M.D.

Figure 6.1: Protocol 1: copies of the first two pages. Protocol kindly provided to the author by Dr. Monica M. Bertagnolli, Chair, Cancer and Acute Leukemia Group B.

Protocol 2

Protocol 2 was carried out under the aegis of the first leukemia group, the Acute Leukemia Group B, now Cancer and Leukemia Group B. Why was it called Group B? Frei and Holland provided the answer. After the first leukemia group was started with three institutions and Protocol 1 was initiated, the Cancer Chemotherapy National Service Center was organized and its Clinical Studies Panel, under Dr. Isidor S. Ravdin (1894-1972), adopted the idea proposed by Zubrod that cooperative oncology groups could be the mechanism of clinical implementation. Burchenal, Frei and Holland were also members of the Clinical Studies Panel. There was a consensus that groups should be organized geographically with Eastern, Central, Southeastern and Southwestern Groups primarily devoted to solid tumors, but two groups for acute leukemia where chemotherapy had already demonstrated some effect. Burchenal was clearly senior to Holland so his proposed pediatric activities were designated Acute Leukemia Group A, whereas the National Cancer Institute-Roswell Park Memorial Institute collaboration with its potential expansion was named Acute Leukemia Group B [2, 5]. The Acute Leukemia Group A later changed its name to the Children's Cancer Cooperative Group A.

The design of Protocol 2 for the Acute Leukemia Group B was a return to the sources, namely Zubrod's initial thought of using combination chemotherapy compared to single agents to determine, among other aims, whether the combination delayed the development of resistance. Patients were randomly allocated to three treatment groups: methotrexate and 6-mercaptopurine in combination; methotrexate alone, or 6-mercaptopurine alone. Those who were treated first with 6-mercaptopurine or methotrexate received the alternate drug whenever no response or disease progression supervened, or improvement short of remission occurred [11]. The rationale for the sequential administration of the single agents was Law's observation in experimental animal leukemia of enhanced sensitivity to 6-mercaptopurine after complete resistance to antifolate, and *vice-versa*, a phenomenon referred to as collateral sensitivity [12]. Both children and adults with acute lymphocytic and acute myelocytic leukemias were entered in the study. In children with acute lymphocytic leukemia, the percentage of complete responses (58%) and the number of long-lasting remissions (longer than 48 weeks) were higher in those receiving the combined treatment. However, median survival was the same in the three groups, a mere nine months. Collateral sensitivity was not observed.

Protocol 2 was important on several grounds. It established for the first time in cancer chemotherapy that two drugs given together were better in terms of objective response than their sequential administration, and introduced the concept that intensification of therapy made a difference in the quality of response.

Protocol 3: A Classic in Oncology

Protocols 1 and 2 investigated means of inducing improved remissions in acute leukemia. Could some drugs be useful in prolonging such remissions? How could their effects be documented, given the situation at the time, with clinical trials of new drugs restricted to patients with advanced disease? The problem was particularly challenging in acute leukemia, where severe complications such as infections and bleeding are common and may cause death before a potentially effective treatment might have time to improve the course of the disease. Freireich with the Acute Leukemia Group B tackled these problems in a study that stands as a leap forward over the obstacles on the road to the cure of cancer. The study design, double-blind and placebo-controlled, had a predecessor, the first ever in cancer treatment, which had been carried out in patients with acute leukemia refractory to 6-mercaptopurine, methotrexate or other antifolates, who also had received at least one course of corticosteroids [13]. In that study, although the new agent was found to have no significant antileukemic activity, it was noted that a proportion of patients in the placebo group showed objective hematologic improvement "which might be ascribed to a prospective new agent [13]". This study which was of importance in the design of Protocol 3, suggested that the potential activity of a new drug would better be studied in patients in remission, and that comparing it to an inactive compound would clearly prove an anticancer effect, if it existed. Before it was accepted, Protocol 3 was hotly debated particularly between Freireich and Holland, who passionately defended their opinions: "When the faces of both would turn red and before things would become out of hand, Frei would say 'Now J' and Dr. Donal Pinkel (see below)

'Now Jim' [14]!" A temporary calm would ensue. Finally the arguments of Dr. Edmund A. Gehan, the group statistician, rallied the investigators to boldly compare the effectiveness of a chemotherapeutic drug and an inactive placebo in a remission maintenance study [15].

But now let's turn to the design of Protocol 3, an Acute Leukemia Group B study of patients under the age of 20 with acute lymphocytic and acute myelocytic leukemias who had received no prior therapy. The study essentially proceeded along an induction and a maintenance phase. Corticosteroids had been shown to produce the highest remission rates in acute leukemia, but these remissions were short lived and not significantly prolonged by maintenance corticosteroid therapy. The corticosteroid selected for the induction phase was prednisone, administered at a dose of 40 mg per square meter of body surface area (mg/sq m). Patients who developed a complete remission within 28 days entered the maintenance phase and were randomly allocated to either 6-mercaptopurine 3 mg per kilogram (mg/kg) daily or to a placebo, both compounds being administered in a double-blind manner: neither the patient, nor the physician knew which compound was given. Maintenance therapy was continued until bone marrow relapse occurred. Patients who did not develop a complete response during the induction phase received 6-mercaptopurine; those who were on the placebo were also treated with the active drug upon relapse. Of the 97 eligible patients, 92 (95%) were analyzed. The results showed a median duration of complete remission of 33 weeks for patients treated with 6-mercaptopurine compared to 9 weeks for those treated with the placebo, a highly significant difference. The median overall survival between the two groups was not significantly different, likely due to the fact that non-responding or relapsing patients were treated with 6-mercaptopurine, and so the fact of being on a placebo did not compromise survival. However, some long-term survivors were seen among patients who received 6-mercaptopurine as maintenance therapy. The study also showed that the best responses to induction therapy, close to 80% complete and partial responses, occurred in children with acute lymphocytic leukemia who were under the age of 15 years.

From a clinical point of view Protocol 3 led to the identification of two separate phases in the treatment of acute leukemia, induction and maintenance, and clearly demonstrated that the antileukemic activity of a drug could be detected by studying the duration of unmaintained remission following remission induction. The demonstrated activity against a tumor that was below the threshold of detection was one of the cornerstones in the rationale for postoperative chemotherapy of solid tumors where clinically undetectable micrometastases might be present. It also became a model for the study of new drugs and made it possible to classify chemotherapeutic agents according to their inducing, maintaining, or inducing-maintaining activity. As was to become apparent, some drugs were more effective in their capacity to induce remissions rather than maintaining them, and *vice-versa*. This study also had a major impact on the development of the design and statistical analysis of clinical trials. In particular, a sequential experimental design was used that made it possible to discontinue the study as soon as a significant difference in duration of the maintenance phase between the two treatment groups was observed. Protocol 3 has been recognized as a landmark clinical trial in a publication that provides details on its background, design, conduct and impact [16].

The reader might well ask why two methods of drug dosage were used, one based on body weight in kilograms and the other on body surface area in square meter. Dr. Donald Pinkel (Fig. **6.2**) from the Department of Pediatrics at Roswell Park Memorial Institute was a member of the Acute Leukemia Group B and had participated in all three protocols described above. As a pediatrician, he was aware that blood levels of many medications used in children are directly related to body surface area. When he began his career as a pediatrician in the cancer field, he noted that the toxicity of a chemotherapeutic drug, dactinomycin, did not correlate at all with body weight, but correlated perfectly with body surface area. This led him to investigate the relationships between cancer drugs and body surface area [14].

In 1958, Pinkel published an important paper reviewing the relationship between a number of physiological functions and body surface area [17]. He showed that the doses of four out of five chemotherapeutic agents were closely similar among rodents, infants, older children and adults when expressed in mg per unit of body surface area, but differed widely when expressed in mg per unit of body weight. For example, the therapeutic dose ratio of methotrexate between the dose in a mouse and the dose in an adult was 21 when expressed in mg per unit of body weight and 1.3 when expressed on the basis of unit per body surface area.

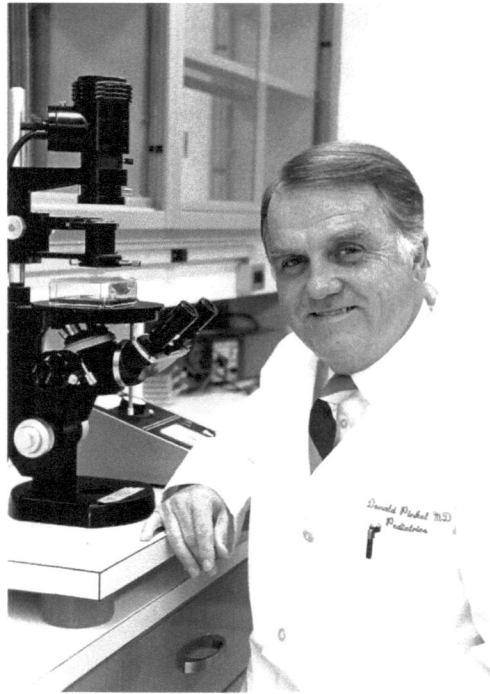

Figure 6.2: Dr. Donald Pinkel. Photograph kindly provided to the author by Dr. Pinkel.

Pinkel concluded his paper by wrinting: "It is suggested that cancer chemotherapists consider the applicability of body surface area as a criterion of drug dosage in their laboratory and clinical studies [17]". In Protocol 3, the only drug given on a body surface area basis was prednisone. According to Pinkel it must have been a concession to him [14]! Later, the administration of chemotherapeutic agents on the basis of body surface area became standard practice.

VINCA ALKALOIDS

In 1952, leaves from the Madagascar periwinkle (*Vinca rosea*), used in Jamaica and in the Philippines as tea to treat diabetes, were provided to Doctors Robert L. Noble (1910-1990) and Charles T. Beer (1915-2010) at the University of Western Ontario in London, Ontario, to extract the active component. Experiments failed to discover an antidiabetic effect; however, the treated animals developed a transient but marked reduction in white blood cell counts. This chance observation eventually led to the discovery of vinblastine, one of the representatives of a new class of anticancer drugs, the vinca alkaloids [18, 19]. Around the same time, Dr. Irving S. Johnson and his colleagues at the Eli Lilly Company in Indianapolis, Indiana, were independently investigating the potential antidiabetic activity of the Madagascar periwinkle. The Canadian and American researchers were unaware of each other's common interest until the program of a New York Academy of Sciences meeting on screening procedures for experimental cancer chemotherapy was announced; both groups met at that conference. Eventually, vinblastine was produced by the Eli Lilly Company. It took about 13,600 kilograms of dried periwinkle leaves to obtain about 28 grams of the drug [19]. From periwinkle extracts, Johnson and his group isolated four compounds with anticancer activity; one of which, vincristine, was active in the P1534 mouse leukemia model but not in the L1210 model [20-22]. "At Eli Lilly, compounds were tested for anticancer activity on a broader screen than that used at the Cancer Chemotherapy National Service Center [22]".

As Freireich recalled, a physician at Eli Lilly who had treated a few cases of lymphoma with vincristine, came to the National Cancer Institute to see whether there was interest in conducting a clinical trial. Since both Zubrod and Frei were out of town, Freireich met the physician and was shown the data. On Frei's return, Freireich indicated his willingness to go ahead. However, Zubrod disagreed because the Acute Leukemia Task Force retrospective study of all drugs active against cancer had established that the L1210 leukemia model was the paradigm for moving from the laboratory to the clinic; vincristine had no effect on L1210, so there was no point in studying it. When Freireich heard this he replied that he had ten dying kids on the ward. "We have nothing else; why not give them the drug?" Frei went back to Zubrod and convinced him that it should be tried. The study revealed that vincristine was highly active in inducing rapid remissions in children with acute leukemia refractory to 6-mercaptopurine and methotrexate, all of whom had also received previous therapy with corticosteroids [23]. "It was unbelievable. It was like magic. We also found that the drug had little effect on the bone marrow and that neurotoxicity was the dose limiting side effect [4]".

There were now four types of non-cross resistant drugs of therapeutic value in childhood acute leukemia: corticosteroids, methotrexate, 6-mercaptopurine and vincristine.

AN INTERLUDE: THE FIRST CANCER CURE

Dr. Min Chiu Li (1919-1980), Fig. **6.3**, was a resident in medicine at Presbyterian Hospital in Chicago, Illinois, before working with Olof Pearson at the Sloan-Kettering Institute for Cancer Research. There, he gave methotrexate to a patient with widespread malignant melanoma and noted that elevated chorionic gonadotropin titers became negative. As Li recounts: "An incidental finding was that, for some strange reason, there was a substantially elevated chorionic gonadotropin titer in the patient's urine . . . It was simply a matter of routine that we did the urinary chorionic gonadotropin assay on a biweekly basis . . . It was this incidental laboratory finding that led me to speculate on the possible therapeutic effect on the chorionic gonadotropin-producing tumors [24]". Trophoblastic tumors are gestational in origin, developing in the placenta and producing high levels of blood and urinary chorionic gonadotropin. The most malignant of these tumors, metastatic chroriocarcinoma, had almost invariably been fatal up to that point.

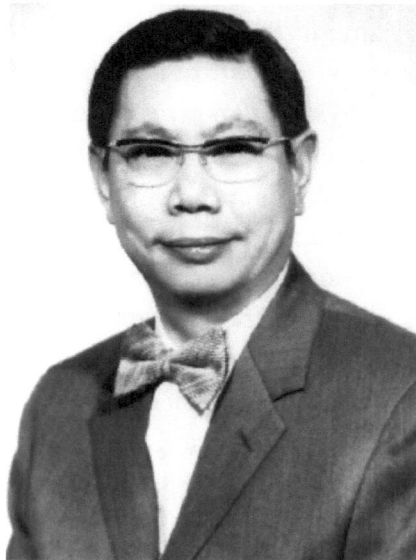

Figure 6.3: Dr. Min Chiu Li. Photograph in: Freireich EJ. Min Chiu Li: a perspective in cancer therapy. Clin Cancer Res 2002; 8:2764-5. Reproduced with permission from the American Association for Cancer Research.

When Li joined the Endocrinology Service of Dr. Roy Hertz (1909-2002) at the National Cancer Institute, he treated women with metastatic choriocarcinoma and other metastatic trophoblastic diseases with intensive intermittent methotrexate until the chorionic gonadotropin titers became normal [25, 26]. These events marked the first cure of a metastatic solid tumor in human subjects. And the cure was derived from a clinician's astute observation that if levels of a biologic marker of viable tumor remain abnormal despite the disappearance of all clinically detectable lesions, then treatment should be pursued until the levels normalize.

VAMP

In November 1962, Freireich initiated a study in childhood acute leukemia with the four chemotherapeutic agents of proven activity available at the time: vincristine, amethopterine (methotrexate), 6-mercaptopurine and prednisone; the study was named VAMP from the first letters of the four drugs. It should be noted, however, that a new drug of a different class, the alkylating agent cyclophosphamide, was reported in October of the same year to induce remissions in children with acute leukemia relapsing after conventional therapy [27]. The purpose of the VAMP trial was to produce the maximum cell-kill, thereby prolonging remission duration. Several considerations influenced the study design. The drugs differed as to their mechanism of action and two of them differed in their dose-limiting toxicity pattern. Skipper and colleagues had shown the first-order kinetic action of chemotherapeutic drugs and the advantage of using high intermittent dosage. Li had demonstrated that to cure choriocarcinoma, treatment needed to be continued beyond the achievement of a complete clinical remission and pursued until the levels of chorionic gonadotropin, reflecting the presence of viable tumor tissue in the body, returned to normal; a median of four courses of methotrexate was needed to achieve these results. Interestingly, autopsy studies of patients with acute leukemia who died while in complete bone marrow remission revealed foci of acute leukemia cells in various organs [28]. Similar findings were obtained in patients alive and in complete remission [29]. The author was working in Mathé's Department at the time, and part of his duties was to perform six bone marrow aspirations at different sites, as well as biopsies of the bone marrow, liver and kidney on these patients.

The VAMP study design therefore included intermittent administration of vincristine and prednisone at full dose, with doses of the other two drugs reduced by one-third due to their hematologic toxicity; five additional courses were given following complete bone marrow remission [30]. "It was quite an emotional experience because almost all the children responded to VAMP quickly, in a week or two. We then treated them with full dose VAMP although they were in complete remission. And this was very dramatic because the parents could not understand why we were doing that. Kids were normal and apparently cured and we were giving treatment that was very toxic. But that turned out to be crucial [4]". It was crucial for a number of reasons. Although the median time to relapse was short, about 22 weeks, two patients remained in complete remission without any treatment for over 22 months. The study pointed to the importance of continuing treatment for longer periods of time beyond the achievement of a complete remission. Application of the fractional cell-kill model to the VAMP study suggested that the data "are consistent with the interpretation that VAMP treatment was indeed effective in reducing the number of leukemic cells to unprecedentedly low levels [31]".

SUPPORTIVE CARE: PLATELETS AND GRANULOCYTE TRANSFUSIONS

Platelet Transfusions

Because of bone marrow replacement of normal hematopoiesis, patients with untreated acute leukemia develop anemia and low platelet counts, as well as low counts of normal granulocytes in the blood despite high counts of leukemic cells. While anemia could be readily corrected with blood transfusions, this was not the case for granulocytes and platelets. In the 1950s, over 50% of deaths from acute leukemia were due to bleeding and/or infections [32]. These problems were compounded by the fact that some of the chemotherapeutic drugs used were hematotoxic, which also led to decreased platelet and granulocyte counts, with the accompanying risk of bleeding and infections. The medical wisdom of the time was that circulating anticoagulants, not low platelet counts, were the main factors and that platelet transfusions alone would not correct the bleeding. In addition, preparation and preservation of platelets for transfusion purposes was fraught with difficulties.

It was under these circumstances that Zubrod made rounds one day with Frei and Freireich. Afterwards, he commented: "This ward is like an abattoir, there is blood on the pillows, on the sheets, on the gowns, there is blood everywhere! Freireich you must do something about this. So like when he asked me to cure leukemia, I said 'Yes Sir'. What was happening is that many children had developed meningeal leukemia which we did not recognize clinically at the time. They were semi-conscious, breathing stertorously, spraying blood from their mouth and nose [4]". Freireich proceeded to conduct laboratory experiments that suggested that platelets were important in the bleeding process of his patients. He then performed an exchange transfusion in a child with acute leukemia who was bleeding and had extremely low platelet counts. Platelet-rich plasma directly obtained from healthy blood donors was used; the platelet count rose from 1,000 per cubic millimetre to about 100,000 per cubic millimetre and the bleeding stopped. However, bleeding recurred when the platelet count fell below 10,000 per cubic millimeter. This convinced Freireich that platelet depletion played an important role in the development of hemorrhage in patients with acute leukemia. He also studied platelets in blood stored in the blood bank and noted that a few days after the date of blood collection, platelets rapidly decreased in number and function. A randomized double-blind study comparing transfusions of fresh blood *versus* blood stored in the blood bank was then carried out in nine patients; the results showed a statistically significant effect of fresh blood in controlling bleeding and in raising platelet counts [33]. Freireich presented the data at a major National Institutes of Health grand rounds attended by clinical and laboratory directors, but the head of clinical laboratory, whose work in experimental animals had shown that platelet depletion did not cause bleeding, rebutted his argument. The conclusion was that fresh blood would not be supplied to Freireich for the treatment of hemorrhage in patients with acute leukemia.

Freireich vividly recalled this event. "At this point, Dr. Zubrod stood-up; Zubrod was a very elegant looking and elegant speaking man; he stood-up in all his majesty, did not go to the stage to address the audience and said in essence: 'I listened to all the data and I conclude as Clinical Director that if my doctors order fresh blood, it is your obligation to comply' [4]". That must have been a very unusual and extraordinary tense meeting as the event was commented upon, more than 25 years later, by both Frei and Zubrod. Frei had written: "For Freireich, myself, and our young colleagues, this courage, this support of younger colleagues in adversity, and this vision of the future had a profound effect [34]". Zubrod added: "These studies (by Dr. Freireich) were vigorously attacked by classical hematologists . . . I recall a dramatic showdown at a clinical staff meeting in 1956 where a motion was made to deny platelets to NCI [35]".

Subsequently, the technique of plasmapheresis was adapted to produce large amounts of platelet-rich plasma. And so, the inverse relationship between platelet counts and bleeding was recognized, leading to the prophylactic use of platelets when platelet counts dropped below 20,000 per cubic millimetre. As a consequence, the major cause of death of patients with acute leukemia was no longer low platelet counts and hemorrhage, but low granulocyte counts and infections [36-39].

Granulocyte Transfusions

Decreased granulocyte counts are the main factor predisposing to bacterial infections in acute leukemia [40]. In Mathé's Department [41] and elsewhere [42] transfusions of granulocytes from patients with chronic myelocytic leukemia were attempted to correct this condition. That approach, although successful, was limited by the availability of donors. Methods of collecting normal granulocytes by whole blood centrifugation were therefore investigated [43, 44]. The development of the method, which now makes possible the routine separation of plasma, red cells and granulocytes from whole blood, faced major technical difficulties that took several years to overcome. The historical development of the continuous-flow blood cell separator and granulocyte transfusions has been informatively related by one of its inventors, Dr. Freireich [45].

With the advent of platelet and granulocyte transfusions, it became possible to control the hemorrhage and infections associated with the disease process of acute leukemia. Equally important, these cellular therapies made it possible to correct the effects of hematotoxic drugs and use increased drug doses with a potential for cure [46, 47].

MENINGEAL LEUKEMIA: AN UNEXPECTED THERAPEUTIC HURDLE

Meningeal leukemia is caused by leukemic cell infiltration of the meninges, giving rise to a clinical syndrome associated with intra-cranial hypertension [48, 49]. Before the advent of chemotherapy, this syndrome was infrequently diagnosed clinically, being eclipsed by the fulminating course of acute leukemia and its associated complications of fever, infection and bleeding. With the increasing frequency and duration of complete hematologic and clinical remissions induced by chemotherapy, meningeal leukemia became the most frequent first evidence of disease recurrence, usually followed by systemic relapse [49, 50].

After therapeutic oral doses of methotrexate, low levels of the drug were found in the spinal fluid; it was inferred that the drug did not penetrate the blood-brain barrier in sufficient concentration [51], a so-called pharmacologic "sanctuary" effect [52]. However, intrathecal administration of methotrexate to four children with acute leukemia produced high drug levels in the spinal fluid and marked symptomatic improvements [51]. These observations "ushered in the whole era of intrathecal MTX (methotrexate) in the treatment and prophylaxis of meningeal leukemia [52]". Other means of treatment and prophylaxis, including radiation therapy of the cranio-spinal axis and other chemotherapeutic agents, were also used [52].

The prevention of meningeal leukemia with prophylactic therapy, first used in an Acute Leukemia Group B controlled clinical trial [52, 53], markedly reduced this complication and prolonged the duration of complete remissions in childhood acute leukemia [54, 55].

PROTECTION FROM DRUG TOXICITY

As noted in the previous chapter, high doses of methotrexate with leucovorin rescue protected against the lethal toxicity of the drug and improved the survival of the treated mice. That observation was directly carried over clinically. Dr. Isaac Djerassi (1925-2111) of the Children's Hospital in Philadelphia, Pennsylvania reported that massive doses of methotrexate exhibited therapeutic effects in childhood acute leukemia and could be safely administered when followed by leucovorin rescue [56]. This technique was later used in the treatment of other malignancies [57-60]. It is interesting to note that this approach was active against tumor "sanctuary" sites not reached in adequate concentrations by standard systemic doses of methotrexate: primary brain cancers [61] and leukemic infiltration of the testes [62].

CLASSICS IN ONCOLOGY: DOSE-SCHEDULE, CONSOLIDATION, PERIODIC REINDUCTION

The Acute Leukemia Group B designed a controlled clinical trial based on Goldin's experimental study showing the superiority of twice weekly methotrexate over daily administration in early leukemia. Children with acute lymphocytic leukemia in remission following induction with vincristine and prednisone were randomly allocated to a maintenance phase consisting of daily or twice-weekly methotrexate. Although the side effects of the two regimens were of similar degree, the dose of methotrexate was three times higher and the duration of complete remission four times longer in children receiving intermittent treatment [63]. This study not only confirmed the importance of the dose-schedule concept in cancer therapy, but radically modified the clinical investigation of new drugs. As it was aptly stated: "The scope of drug trials has been enormously amplified, each agent becoming in practice many agents, dependent upon its mode of administration [64]".

In 1966, the Acute Leukemia Group B initiated a new study, ALGB study 6601, a clinical trial in 325 children with acute leukemia. After an induction phase using vincristine and prednisone, children in complete remission were randomly allocated to a consolidation phase consisting of three different dose levels of methotrexate. This was followed by a second randomization into a four-arm maintenance phase. Group one received no further therapy, while groups two and three were treated twice-weekly with methotrexate at two different dose levels and also received periodic intrathecal instillation of the drug. In group four, regimen D, periodic reinduction with vincristine and prednisone, the same agents used during the induction phase, were added to twice-weekly methotrexate; intrathecal methotrexate was also given. After eight months of study, two groups, including regimen D, were randomized to no further therapy or twice-weekly methotrexate for an additional indefinite time period. Remission induction was achieved in 85% of the children. The best results were obtained in regimen D, with almost one-quarter of children remaining in complete remission four years or longer after completion of therapy [54, 65, 66].

The integration of the new concepts of consolidation and periodic reinduction into the concepts of induction, maintenance, central nervous system prophylactic therapy and longer trial duration, has established principles of chemotherapy that remain the pillars of current treatment for childhood acute leukemia.

Pinkel at St. Jude Children's Research Hospital in Memphis, Tennessee, used a somewhat similar approach but with continuous multidrug therapy for two to three years, a program referred to as "total therapy" [67]. In studies initiated between 1962 and 1965, seven of 37 children (19 %) with acute leukemia remained in complete remission, off therapy, for nine or more years [67-69].

These extraordinary achievements of rigorous clinical trials, derived in part from pre-clinical experimental data [70], contrast markedly with the four-month median survival from diagnosis to death in untreated childhood acute leukemia [71].

REFERENCES

[1]   Gilman A. The initial clinical trial of nitrogen mustard. Am J Surg 1963; 105:574-8.
[2]   Author's interview with Dr. Emil Frei III.
[3]   Author's interview with Dr. Bayard Clarkson.
[4]   Author's interview with Dr. Emil J. Freireich.
[5]   Author's interview with Dr. James F. Holland.
[6]   Bisel HF. Criteria for the evaluation of response to treatment in acute leukemia. Blood 1956; 11:676-7.
[7]   Frei E III, Holland JF, Schneiderman MA, *et al.* A comparative study of two regimens of combination chemotherapy in acute leukemia. Blood 1958; 13:1126-48.
[8]   Streptomycin treatment of pulmonary tuberculosis: a Medical Research Council investigation. Br Med J 1948; 2:769-82.
[9]   Hill AB. Suspended judgment. Memories of the British streptomycin trial in tuberculosis. The first randomized clinical trial. Control Clin Trials 1990; 11:77-9.
[10]   Armitage P. Fisher, Bradford Hill, and randomisation. Int J Epidemiol 2003; 32:925-8.
[11]   Frei E III, Freireich EJ, Gehan E, *et al.* Studies of sequential and combination antimetabolite therapy in acute leukemia: 6-mercaptopurine and methotrexate. Blood 1961; 18:431-54.
[12]   Law LW. Differences between cancers in terms of evolution of drug resistance. Cancer Res 1956; 16:698-716.
[13]   Freireich EJ, Frei E III, Holland JF, *et al.* Evaluation of new chemotherapeutic agent in patients with ⬚ advanced refractory⬚ acute leukemia. Studies of 6-azauracil. Blood 1960; 16:1268-1278.
[14]   Author's interview with Dr. Donald Pinkel.
[15]   Freireich EJ, Gehan E, Frei E III, *et al.* The effect of 6-Mercaptopurine on the duration of steroid-induced remissions in acute leukemia: a model for evaluation of other potentially useful therapy. Blood 1963; 21:699-716.

[16]   Gehan EA, Freireich EJ. The 6-MP *versus* placebo clinical trial in acute leukemia. Clin Trials 2011; 8:288-297.

[17]   Pinkel D. The use of body surface area as a criterion of drug dosage in cancer chemotherapy. Cancer Res 1958; 18:853-6.

[18]   Noble RL, Beer CT, Cutts JH. Role of chance observations in chemotherapy: *vinca rosea*. Ann NY Acad Sci 1958; 76:882-94.

[19]   Noble RL. The discovery of the vinca alkaloids --chemotherapeutic agents against cancer. Biochem Cell Biol 1990; 68:1344-51.

[20]   Johnson IS, Wright HF, Svoboda GH. Experimental basis for clinical evaluation of antitumor principles derived from *Vinca rosea* Linn. J Lab Clin Med 1959: 54:830.

[21]   Johnson IS, Armstrong JG, Gorman M, Burnett JP Jr. The vinca alkaloids: a new class of oncolytic agents. Cancer Res 1963; 23:1390-1427.

[22]   Author's interview with Dr. Irving S Johnson.

[23]   Karon MR, Freireich EJ, Frei E. A preliminary report on vincristine sulphate-a new active agent for the treatment of acute leukemia. Pediatrics 1962; 30:791-6.

[24]   Li MC. *Discussion of the paper*: Chemotherapy of choriocarcinoma and related trophoblastic tumors in women by Hertz R, Bergenstal DM, Lippsett MB, Price EB, Hilbish TF. Ann NY Acad Sci 1959; 80:262-84.

[25]   Li MC, Hertz R, Spencer DB. Effect of methotrexate therapy upon choriocarcinoma and chorioadenoma. Proc Soc Exp Biol Med 1956; 93:361-6.

[26]   Li MC, Hertz R, Bergenstal DM. Therapy of choriocarcinoma and related trophoblastic tumors with folic acid and purine antagonists. N Engl J Med 1958; 259:66-74.

[27]   Fernbach DJ, Sutow WW, Thurman WG, Vietti TJ. Clinical evaluation of cyclophosphamide. A new agent for the treatment of children with acute leukemia. JAMA 1962; 182:30-7.

[28]   Nies BA, Bodey GP, Thomas LB, Brecher G, Freireich EJ. The persistence of extramedullary leukemic infiltrates during bone marrow remission of acute leukemia. Blood 1965; 26:133-41.

[29]   Mathé G, Schwarzenberg L, Mery AM, *et al.* Extensive histological and cytological survey of patients with acute leukemia in "complete remission". Br Med J 1966; 1:640-2.

[30]   Freireich EJ, Karon M, Frei E 3rd. Quadruple combination therapy (VAMP) for acute lymphocytic leukemia of childhood. Proc Am Assoc Cancer Res 1964; 5:20.

[31]   Frei E 3rd, Freireich EJ. Progress and perspectives in the chemotherapy of acute leukemia. Adv Chemother 1965; 2:269-98.

[32]   Hersh EM, Bodey GP, Nies BA, Freireich EJ. Causes of death in acute leukemia: A ten-year study of 414 patients from 1954-1963. JAMA 1965; 193:105-9.

[33]   Freireich EJ, Schmidt PJ, Schneiderman MA, Frei E 3rd. A comparative study of the effect of transfusion of fresh and preserved whole blood on bleeding in patients with acute leukemia. N Engl J Med 1959; 260:6-11.

[34]   Frei E III. Confrontation, passion, and personalization. Emil J Freireich. Clin Cancer Res 1997; 3 (12Pt 2):2554-62.

[35]   Zubrod CG. Origins and development of chemotherapy research at the National Cancer Institute. Cancer Treat Rep 1984; 68:9-19.

[36]   Kliman A, Gaydos LA, Schroeder LR, Freireich EJ. Repeated plasmapheresis of blood donors as a source of platelets. Blood 1961; 18:303-9.

[37]   Gaydos LA, Freireich EJ, Mantel N. The quantitative relation between platelet count and hemorrahge in patients with acute leukemia. N Engl J Med 1962; 266:905-9.

[38]   Freireich EJ, Kliman A, Gaydos LA, Mantel N, Frei E 3rd. Response to repeated platelet transfusion from the same donor. Ann Int Med 1963; 59:277-87.

[39]   Freireich EJ. Origins of platelet transfusion therapy. Transfus Med Rev 2011; 25:252-6.

[40]   Bodey GP, Buckley M, Sathe YS, Freireich EJ. Quantitative relationships between circulating leukoctes and infection in patients with acute leukemia. Ann Intern Med 1966; 64:328-40.

[41]   Schwarzenberg L, Mathé G, De Grouchy J, *et al.* White blood cell transfusions. Israel J Med Sci 1965; 1:925-56.

[42]   Morse EE, Freireich EJ, Carbone PP, Bronson W, Frei E. The transfusion of leukocytes from donors with chronic myelocytic leukemia to patients with leucopenia. Transfusion 1966; 6:183-92.

[43]   Freireich EJ, Judson G, Levin RH. Separation and collection of leukocytes. Cancer Res 1965; 25:1516-20.

[44]   Judson G, Jones A, Kellogg R, *et al.* Closed continuous-flow centrifuge. Nature 1968; 217: 816-8.

[45]   Freireich EJ. Leukocyte transfusion and the development of the continuous-flow blood cell separator. Transfus Med Rev 2011; 25:344-50.

[46]   Schwarzenberg L, Mathé G. White cell transfusions: six years experience. Br J Haematol 1969; 17:603-4.

[47]   Simone JV. Use of fresh blood components during intensive combination therapy of childhood leukemia. Cancer 1971; 28:562-5.

[48]   Moore EW, Thomas LB, Shaw RK, Freireich EJ. The central nervous system in acute leukemia: a postmortem study of 117 consecutive cases, with particular reference to hemorrhages, leukemic infiltrations and the syndrome of meningeal leukemia. Arch Intern Med 1960; 105:451-68.

[49]   Shaw RK, Moore EW, Freireich EJ, Thomas LB. Meningeal leukemia: A syndrome resulting from increased intracranial pressure in patients with acute leukemia. Neurology 1960; 10:823-33.

[50]   Evans AE, Gilbert ES, Zandstra R. The increasing incidence of central nervous system leukemia in children (Children's Cancer Study Group A). Cancer 1970; 26:404-9.

[51]   Whiteside JA, Philips FS, Dargeon HW, Burchenal JH. Intrathecal amethopterin in neurological manifestations of leukemia. Arch Intern Med 1958; 101:279-85.

[52]   Burchenal JH. History of intrathecal prophylaxis and therapy of meningeal leukemia. Cancer Drug Deliv 1983; 1:87-92.

[53]   Frei E III, Karon M, Levin RH, *et al.* The effectiveness of combinations of antileukemic agents in inducing and maintaining remission in children with acute leukemia. Blood 1965; 26:642-56.

[54]   Holland JF. *E Pluribus Unum*: Presidential Address. Cancer Res 1971; 31:1319-29.

[55]   Aur RJ, Simone J, Hustu HO, *et al.* Central nervous system therapy and combination chemotherapy of childhood lymphocytic leukemia. Blood 1971; 37:272-81.

[56]   Djerassi I, Abir E, Royer GL Jr, Treat CL. Long-term remissions in childhood acute leukemia: use of infrequent infusions of methotrexate; supportive roles of platelet transfusions and citrovorum factor. Clin Pediatr 1966; 5:502-9.

[57]   Djerassi I, Kim JS. Methotrexate and citrovorum factor rescue in the management of childhood lymphosarcoma and reticulum cell sarcoma (non-Hodgkin's lymphomas): prolonged unmaintained remissions. Cancer 1976; 38:1043-51.

[58]   Ambinder EP, Perloff M, Ohnuma T, Biller HF, Holland JF. High dose methotrexate followed by citrovorum factor reversal in patients with advanced cancer. Cancer 1979; 43:1177-82.

[59]   Frei E 3rd, Blum RH, Pitman SW, *et al*. High dose methotrexate with leucovorin rescue. Rationale and spectrum of antitumor activity. Am J Med 1980; 68:370-6.

[60]   Reggev A, Djerassi I. The safety of administration of massive doses of methotrexate (50 g) with equimolar citrovorum factor rescue in adult patients. Cancer 1988; 61:2423-8.

[61]   Djerassi I, Kim JS, Reggev A. Response of astrocytoma to high-dose methotrexate with citrovorum factor rescue. Cancer 1985; 55:2741-7.

[62]   Brecher ML, Weinberg V, Boyett JM, *et al*. Intermediate dose methotrexate in childhood acute lymphoblastic leukemia resulting in decreased incidence of testicular relapse. Cancer 1986; 58:1024-8.

[63]   New treatment schedule with improved survival in childhood leukemia: Intermittent parenteral *vs* daily oral administration of methotrexate for maintenance of induced remission. Acute Leukemia Group B. JAMA 1965; 194:75-81.

[64]   Henderson ES. Treatment of acute leukemia. Ann Intern Med 1968; 69:628-32.

[65]   Holland JF, Glidewell O. Chemotherapy of acute lymphocytic leukemia of childhood. Cancer 1972; 30:1480-7.

[66]   Holland JF. Combination therapy of acute lymphocytic leukemia of children. JAMA 1972; 222:1169-70.

[67]   Pinkel D. Five-year follow-up of "total therapy" of childhood lymphocytic leukemia. JAMA 1971; 216:648-52.

[68]   Pinkel D. Total therapy of acute lymphocytic leukemia. JAMA 1972; 222:1170.

[69]   Pinkel D. The ninth annual David Karnofsky Lecture. Treatment of acute lymphocytic leukemia. Cancer 1979; 43:1128-37.

[70]   Goldin A. Pre-clinical chemotherapy: historical aspects. Mt Sinai J Med 1985; 52:419-25.

[71]   Tivey H. The natural history of untreated acute leukemia. Ann NY Acad Sci 1954; 60:322-58.

Therapeutic Revolution, 2014, 85-93

"The medical profession has a responsibility not only for the cure of the sick and for the prevention of disease but for the advancement of knowledge upon which both depend. This third responsibility can be met only by investigation and experiment".
Dr. Robert A. McCance.

CHAPTER 7

The Years of Creativity: 1953-1965. Cooperative Oncology Groups and Clinical Trials

Pierre R. Band[*]

Department of Medicine, McGill University, Montreal, Canada

Abstract: Cooperative oncology groups were formed by the Cancer Chemotherapy National Service Center to test on humans promising chemotherapeutic drugs that were coming through the screening program. Patients from several institutions were pooled to shorten the time required to test new compounds against various malignancies, establish standards and objective criteria for diagnosis, patient selection, treatment and measurement of effect, and ensure statistically valid study designs and data analyses. The different phases of clinical investigation of malignant tumors were created: Phase I to establish the maximal tolerated dose of the new agent, its toxicity and pattern of reversibility; Phase II to look for activity in a broad spectrum of malignancies, which required the elaboration of objective criteria for therapeutic response; and Phase III to determine the efficacy and safety of the new drug in the specific cancer sites where activity had been observed in a Phase II study.

Keywords: Cooperative oncology groups, Phase I, Phase II, Phase III.

INTRODUCTION

In the preceding chapter we saw that Protocol 1 was the first cooperative study of a human malignancy undertaken by investigators from three different institutions, while Protocol 2 was carried out by the Acute Leukemia Group B. The Cancer Chemotherapy National Service Center and its Clinical Studies Panel formed the cooperative oncology groups to test on human cancers new chemotherapeutic drugs that had been developed through the screening program. Groups were

---

*Address correspondence to Pierre R. Band: Faculty of Medicine, McGill University, Montreal, Quebec H3G 1Y6, Canada; E-mail: pierre.band@gmail.com

formed to pool patients from several institutions in order to shorten the time required to test new agents against various malignancies, establish standards and objective criteria for diagnosis, patient selection, treatment and measurement of effect, and ensure statistically valid study designs and data analyses [1]. In addition, it was hoped that the information gained would "provide a basis for correlation with animal studies in order to find those animal systems that have a high predicting value for effectiveness in human tumors [2]". A major and insufficiently emphasized benefit of these endeavours has been improvement in the quality of care for cancer patients. The Eastern Solid Tumor Group (ESTG), later called the Eastern Cooperative Oncology Group (ECOG), which was organized to study the effect of drugs against solid tumors, and the Acute Leukemia Group B (ALGB), later called the Cancer and Leukemia Group B, were the first groups to be created, in 1955; by the end of the decade 18 cooperative oncology groups had been formed across the United States [1].

The ESTG's first study was a comparative clinical trial of two anticancer drugs in patients with lung cancer, breast cancer, malignant melanoma and Hodgkin's disease. The main purposes, as may be inferred from the publication's title, were not so much to assess the effectiveness of the drugs, as to "study the feasibility and usefulness of collaborative clinical research in cancer chemotherapy", "apply known principles of the therapeutic trial to clinical cancer chemotherapy", and "develop useful quantitative measures of antitumor effects of drugs upon human solid tumors [3]". In addition to defining objective criteria for the various protocol parameters, this study also introduced a five-step performance status scale that was simpler than the ten-step Karnofsky scale [4]. This new scale, known as Zubrod's or the ECOG performance status is shown in Table **7.1** as originally reported [3].

It is important to bear in mind that the initial studies by the ALGB and the ESTG were not what would today be considered Phase III studies.

Table 7.1: Eastern Cooperative Oncology Group: Performance Status

Grade	Performance Status
0	Normal activities
1	Symptoms, but nearly fully ambulatory
2	Some bed time, but needs to be in bed less than 50 % of normal day time
3	Needs to be in bed greater than 50% of normal daytime
4	Unable to get out of bed

"At the beginning, what prevailed was the importance of biostatistically relevant conclusions. It was clearly Zubrod who advanced the concept of the randomized clinical trial in oncology and the need to get adequate numbers of patients to make statistically valid decisions. The concept of Phase I, II and III evolved from that [5]". Indeed, the first mention of the different phases of clinical trial came later. "In order to clarify various developmental aspects of clinical cancer chemotherapy drug trials, certain terms have been developed. A Phase I study indicates an investigation into the clinical pharmacology and toxicology of any specific new agent. Phase II is a study of the therapeutic response, optimum dosage regimen and best route of administration for any single agent. The Phase III study is a definitive trial comparing, in general, two or possibly more agents in a single disease [1]". These principles of prime importance were adopted in the United States by the Food and Drug Administration in 1962 [6]. Freireich clarified the background to this terminology:

> At the meetings of the Acute Leukemia Task Force, new agents under study were discussed and it was realized that all drugs were started at very low dose and were dropped if no responses were observed. We began to appreciate that we did not really know if the drugs were truly inactive because they were not pursued to the maximum tolerated dose and we realized that we might be overlooking active compounds. This was the basis for separating the first evaluation of the drug, its toxicity and reversibility pattern, from the evaluation of its effectiveness which led to the concepts of Phase I and Phase II [7].

Now let's take a closer look at how these concepts were put in concrete form.

PHASE I STUDIES

Once a drug passed the hurdles of pre-clinical studies showing promise for potential clinical activity, it entered the field of human experimentation. The main purposes of a Phase I study were to establish the maximum tolerated dose of the new agent, the toxicity and reversibility patterns of the drug, and its clinical pharmacology. Patients offered participation in Phase I studies had to have advanced disease refractory to standard therapy and a life expectancy of at least two months. Since antitumor activity was not an essential part of this first phase of clinical drug trial, measurable tumors were not required. At the beginning of a Phase I study, the clinical investigator had knowledge of the maximum tolerated dose and the toxicity of the drug in various animal species. With respect to the latter, it was shown that the predictive value of toxic effects was relatively good for bone marrow, gastrointestinal tract, liver and kidney, questionable for the nervous system, and worthless for the skin and appendages [8]. Hence, the clinical investigator needed to remain alert to unexpected untoward reactions. But what about the very first dose to be administered safely to patients? It was found empirically that a safe dose could be derived from the maximum tolerated dose given over a two-week period to the most susceptible animal species. Accordingly, one proposal was to initiate a Phase I clinical trial using 1/10th that dose on a mg/kg basis for a specified number of days with, thereafter and in the same patient, cautiously increasing the dose levels in a stepwise manner until reversible side effects occurred [9]. Other starting dose recommendations were also proposed [10].

To bring a more coherent approach to the methodology of Phase I studies, the Midwest Cooperative Chemotherapy Group described a new procedure for determining the maximum tolerated dose. All patients treated at a given dose level received the same dose for a fixed number of days. The initial dose was 1/100th of the acute lethal dose that killed 50 % of dogs, administered on a mg/kg basis. If no toxicity supervened, this dose was subsequently doubled in a geometric progression in different groups of patients until toxicity was observed; the dose was then modulated until the highest non-toxic dose was reached [10]. Because the two-fold level increments could suddenly lead to intolerable or irreversible toxicity (Fig. **7.1**), a different method, referred to as the modified Fibonacci search scheme, was developed, using dose escalation levels in progressively decreasing steps to minimize the risk of severe side effects [11]. In a Fibonacci series, the first two numbers are 0 and 1 and each successive number is the sum of the two previous ones; thus: 0, 1, 1, 2, 3, 5, 8, 13, 21 and so forth. Only the number 2 represents a doubling (100% increase) over the previous number; all subsequent numbers are less than double the previous ones. In the modified Fibonacci search scheme, the percentage increase did not exactly follow the increases in a Fibonacci series. Increasing doses for Phase I studies have used percentage increments of 100%, 66%, 50% and 30% to 35% thereafter until the maximum tolerated dose was reached, or similar stepwise increments [11, 12].

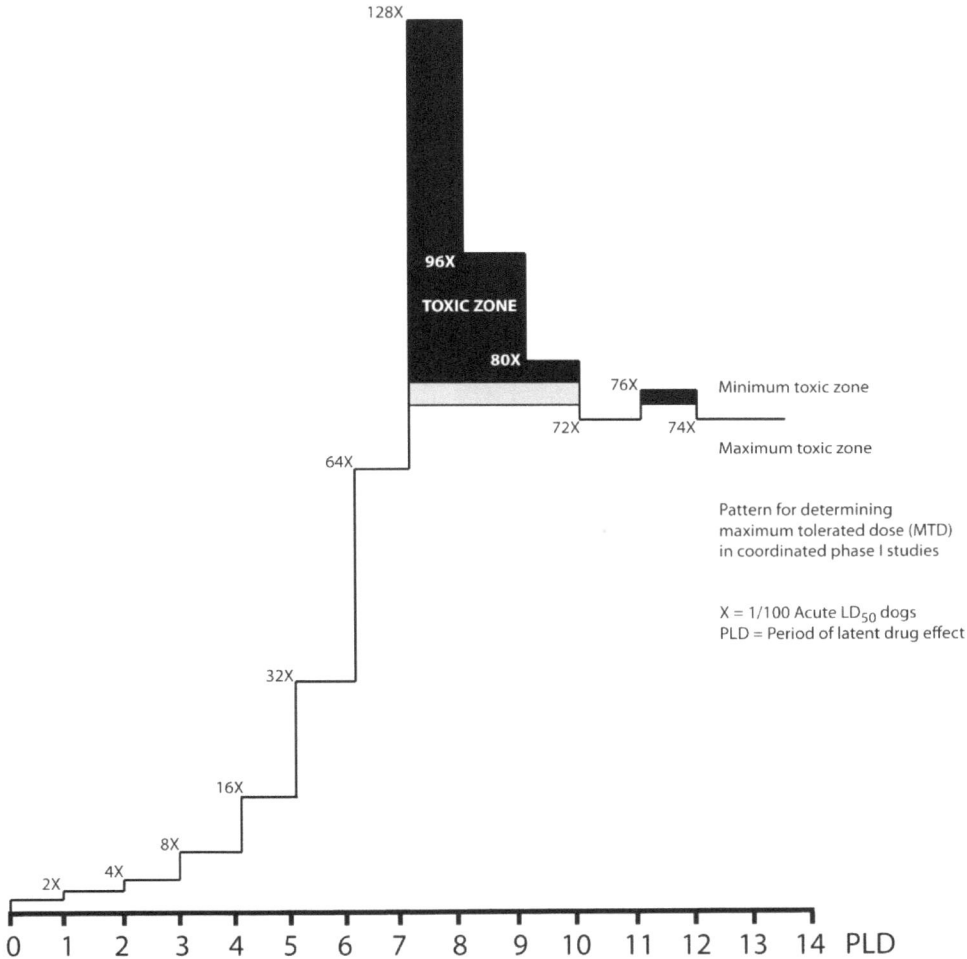

Figure 7.1: Procedure suggested to determine the maximal tolerated dose in Phase I studies. Fig. 1, page 276 in: Louis J. Coordinated Phase I studies for cooperative chemotherapy groups. J. Chron Dis 1962; 15:173-81, reference 10. Reproduced with permission from Elsevier.

Extensive data obtained for 18 anticancer agents were evaluated to determine whether there was a correlation for toxicologic endpoints between animals of various species and man. It was observed that the maximum tolerated dose of a chemotherapeutic drug in humans was closely related to the dose in experimental animals when dosage was expressed based on body surface area [13]. These results provided guidelines for the initial dose to be administered in Phase I clinical trials. In general, a safe initial dose was found to be one-third the maximum tolerated dose in milligrams per square meter of body surface area in the most sensitive animal species [14].

PHASE II STUDIES

The aim of Phase II studies was to demonstrate reproducible clinical activity of new drugs in as broad a spectrum of human malignancies as feasible. The main requirement was the presence of measurable disease to assess drug effect objectively. The ESTG became an innovator in the field of solid tumor clinical trials by using serial measurements of tumor size to assess therapeutic activity and introducing criteria for tumor response and progression [14]. Tumor masses were measured with callipers in two dimensions, the largest tumor diameter and the largest diameter perpendicular to it; the product of these two diameters represented the baseline measurement [14, 15]. However, the percentage decrease or increase in tumor size qualifying respectively for response and progression was not specified [14]. Quantitative response criteria for solid tumors (Table **7.2**) were established in the mid-1960s [16]; widely used, they became known as the ECOG criteria and, with some added minor modifications, have been adopted by the World Health Organization [17].

Table 7.2: Eastern Cooperative Oncology Group: Response Criteria for Solid Tumors. Adapted from [16].

Complete response	Complete disappearance of all measurable lesions
Partial response	Decrease in the sum of the product of tumor diameters by $\geq 50\%$ over two consecutive measurements periods
No change	Decrease of $< 50\%$ of the sum of the product of diameters and an increase of $< 125\%$ over the original measurements
Progression	Increase of $\geq 125\%$ over the original measurements

One of the early issues faced was the sample size needed to decide whether drugs undergoing Phase II studies were likely to have some degree of activity at the dose-schedule used to warrant further studies or were unlikely to be effective. In a seminal paper, Gehan described a statistical approach to the sample size required for a Phase II study. For instance, if we consider a drug to induce a therapeutic effect in 20% of patients with a specific cancer, we would expect at least one response in 14 consecutive patients; in such a case, it was suggested that additional patients be treated to estimate the effectiveness of the drug more precisely. Should there be a zero response, the drug would be unlikely to be active in 20% of the cases and could be dropped with less than a 5% chance of rejecting an active drug [18]. Gehan's plans have largely been followed in clinical trials of Phase II cancer chemotherapeutic agents.

Since Phase II trials for any given cancer site required a minimum of 14 patients with measurable tumor lesions, it was not feasible to conduct Phase II studies in the entire spectrum of human malignancies. Attention was therefore initially focussed on six signal tumors: breast, colon and lung cancers; undifferentiated lymphosarcoma, acute lymphocytic and acute myelocytic leukemias [19]. Prostate cancer, one of the four main solid tumors, was omitted because of the difficulty in measuring bone changes. Phase III studies were then considered for the signal tumors in which Phase II trials demonstrated a drug effect. The initial six signal tumors were subsequently expanded to include other cancer sites [20].

PHASE III STUDIES

A Phase III study may be regarded as the classical clinical trial. Its major objectives are to determine the therapeutic usefulness and safety of the new drug in the specific cancer sites where activity was observed in a Phase II study. It is a major undertaking that necessitates a large number of patients and so is eminently suited to studies carried out by cooperative oncology groups. "The essence of such trial is comparative [21]". The new drug is compared to the standard treatment or to a placebo when there is no standard treatment; of course, with the development of cancer medicine, Phase III studies have surpassed these early aims in design and complexity. Phase III studies involve key statistical procedures such as patient stratification into more homogeneous groups (for instance pre and postmenopausal women), random allocation to treatment groups in order to eliminate investigator bias, and statistical analyses of the data to ensure the clinical validity of the results [21, 22]. Phase III clinical trials establish for a specific cancer the effectiveness of the new drug or therapeutic regimen, which then potentially becomes generally available for the treatment of patients with that specific cancer type.

REFERENCES

[1]   Review of the Cancer Chemotherapy National Service Center program. Cancer Chemother Rep 1959-60; 7:25-46.
[2]   Endicott KM. The chemotherapy program. J Natl Cancer Inst 1957; 19:275-93.
[3]   Zubrod CG, Schneiderman M, Frei E III, *et al.* Appraisal of methods for the study of chemotherapy of cancer in man: comparative therapeutic trial of nitrogen mustard and triethylene thiophosphoramide. J Chron Dis 1960; 11:7-33.
[4]   Karnofsky DA, Burchenal JH. The clinical evaluation of chemotherapeutic agents in cancer. New York: Columbia University Press, 1949. pp. 191-205.
[5]   Author's interview with Dr. James F. Holland.
[6]   Hafkenschiel JH. Government regulations and the use of drugs. Calif Med 1967; 107:159-63.
[7]   Author's interview with Dr. Emil J. Freireich.
[8]   Owens AH Jr. Predicting anticancer drug effects in man from laboratory animal studies. J Chron Dis 1962; 15:223-8.
[9]   Zubrod CG. Clinical investigations in cancer chemotherapy. J Chron Dis 1958; 8:183-90.
[10]   Louis J. Coordinated phase I studies for cooperative chemotherapy groups. J Chron Dis 1962; 15:273-81.
[11]   Carter SK, Selawry O, Slavik M. Phase I clinical trials. Natl Cancer Inst Monogr 1977; 45:75-80.
[12]   Hansen HH., Selawry OS, Muggia FM, Walker MD. Clinical studies with 1-(2-hloroethyl)-3-cyclohexyl-1-nitrosourea (NSC 79037). Cancer Res 1971; 31:223-7.
[13]   Freireich EJ, Gehan EA, Rall DP, Schmidt LH, Skipper HE. Quantitative comparison of toxicity of anticancer agents in mouse, rat, hamster, dog, monkey, and man. Cancer Chemother Rep 1966; 50:219-44.
[14]   Zubrod CG. Multiclinic trials in cancer chemotherapy. CMAJ 1967; 97:101-3.
[15]   Brindley CO, Markoff E, Schneiderman MA. Direct observation of lesion size and number as a method of following the growth of human tumors. Cancer 1959; 12:139-46.
[16]   Carbone PP, Spurr C, Schneiderman M, Scotto J, Holland JF, Shnider B. Management of patients with malignant lymphoma: a comparative study with cyclophosphamide and vinca alkaloids. Cancer Res 1968; 28:811-22.
[17]   Miller AB, Hoogstraten B, Staquet M, Winkler A. Reporting results of cancer treatment. Cancer 1981; 47:207-14.
[18]   Gehan EA. The determination of the number of patients required in a preliminary and a follow-up trial of a new chemotherapeutic agent. J Chronic Dis 1961; 13:346-53.
[19]   Carter SK. The search for therapeutic cell controls by the chemotherapy program of the National Cancer Institute. J Invest Dermatol 1972; 59:128-38.

[20]   Carter SK. Current therapy approaches of the Division of Cancer Treatment with emphasis on pancreatic carcinoma. J Surg Oncol 1974; 6:9-17.

[21]   Hill AB. The clinical trial. New England J Med 1952; 247:113-9.

[22]   Lasagna L. The controlled clinical trial: theory and practice. J Chronic Dis 1955; 1:353-67.

"Combination chemotherapy has been the key to most of the major triumphs for drug treatment". Dr. Steven K. Carter.

CHAPTER 8

Combination Chemotherapy: The Road to Cure

Pierre R. Band[*]

Department of Medicine, McGill University, Montreal, Canada

Abstract: The principles of combination chemotherapy to overcome drug resistance and the use of high intermittent dosage to achieve maximal therapeutic benefits, first learned from studies in childhood acute lymphocytic leukemia, were applied to other hematologic malignancies and to solid tumors. As new drugs that were active against specific malignancies became available, they were tested in combination with other agents. Drugs with different mechanisms of action and no overlapping toxicity were preferentially selected for combination chemotherapy. Cures were achieved in Hodgkin's disease, testicular cancer and Burkitt's lymphoma, as well as improved survival in non-Hodgkin's lymphomas. These major successes occurred in tumors characterized by a relatively rapid proliferating growth rates and were not paralleled by similar results in cancers with slower growth rates.

Keywords: Combination chemotherapy, Hodgkin's disease, non-Hodgkin's lymphomas, Burkitt's lymphoma, testicular cancer, tumor growth rate.

INTRODUCTION

Principles learned from studies carried out in childhood acute lymphocytic leukemia, particularly the importance of combination chemotherapy, were applied to other hematologic malignancies and solid tumors as new agents that were active against specific cancers became available. A number of single agents active against various malignancies were developed between the time the first results were obtained with nitrogen mustard and aminopterin and the early 1970s, when the specialty of medical oncology was created. These agents and the main malignancies against which they have demonstrated activity are shown in Tables **8.1** to **8.3**. A detailed discussion of these drugs may be found in any pharmacology or oncology textbook.

---

*Address correspondence to Pierre R. Band: Faculty of Medicine, McGill University, Montreal, Quebec H3G 1Y6, Canada; E-mail: pierre.band@gmail.com

Table 8.1: Some Single Drugs Active Against Various Malignancies (1940-1975). An International Contribution.

Drugs	Origin
Alkylating Agents	United Kingdom
Busulfan	United Kingdom
Chlorambucil	Germany
Dibromomannitol	Hungary
Melphalan	United Kingdom
Mechlorethamine	United States
Animetabolites	
Cytarabine	United States
Fluororacil	United States
Mercaptopurine	United States
Methotrexate	United States
Mitotic Inhibitors	
Vinbastine	Canada
Vincristine	United States
Antibiotics	
Bleomycin	Japan
Dactinomycin	United States
Daunorubicin	Italy
Doxorubicin	Italy
Other	
L-Asparaginase	United States
Carmustine	United States
Cisplatin	United States
Hydroxyurea	Germany
Dacarbazine	United States
Procarbazine	Switzerland

COMBINATION CHEMOTHERAPY

The background to combination chemotherapy in hematologic malignancies was derived in part from the work of Skipper and colleagues involving the administration of drugs at the maximum tolerated dose to obtain maximal therapeutic benefits, and also Law's work pointing to the use of multiple drugs in an attempt to overcome drug resistance. Results from Freireich's VAMP study and the ALGB in childhood acute leukemia were also drawn upon for the design of drug combination regimens that were likely to lead to improved results over single agents in specific cancers. While the use of single agents was based on activity in experimental animal screening systems, combination chemotherapy was developed on an empiric and pragmatic basis: 1) Drugs that were most active by themselves against a specific malignancy and with different mechanisms of action were preferentially selected; 2) Drugs with no overlapping toxicity were chosen to allow for administration at the maximum tolerated doses; 3) If drugs with overlapping toxicity were included, their doses were reduced to a level commensurate with the dose-limiting toxicity of the combination.

Table 8.2: Some Single Drugs with Main Activity in Indicated Hematologic Malignancies (1940-1975).

Drugs	Cancer	References
Alkylating Agents		
Busulfan	CML	[1]
Chlorambucil	CLL	[2]
Cyclophosphamide	ALL, HD, NHL, Burkitt's Lymphoma	[3-5]
Dibromomannitol	CML	[6]
Mechlorethamine	HD, NHL	[8]
Melphalan	Multiple myeloma	[7]
Antimetabolites		
Cytarabine	ALL, AML	[9-11]
Mercaptopurine	ALL, AML	[11]
Methotrexate	ALL, Burkitt's lymphoma	[11, 12]
Mitotic inhibitors		
Vinblastine	HD, NHL	[13-15]
Vincristine	ALL, AML, HD, Burkitt's lymphoma	[11, 13, 15, 16]
Antibiotics		
Bleomycin	HD, NHL	[17]
Daunorubicin	ALL, AML	[18-20]
Doxorubicin	ALL, AML, HD, NHL	[21]
Other		
L-Asparaginase	ALL	[22]
Carmustine	HD, NHL, Multiple myeloma	[23]
Dacarbazine	HD	[24]
Hydroxyurea	CML	[25]
Procarbazine	HD, NHL	[14, 26]

ALL: acute lymphocytic leukemia; AML: acute myelocytic leukemia; CLL: chronic lymphocytic leukemia; CML: chronic myelocytic leukemia; HD: Hodgkin's disease; NHL: non-Hodgkin's lymphoma.

Table 8.3: Some Single Drugs with Main Activity in Indicated Solid Tumors (1940-1975).

Drugs	Cancer	References
Alkylating Agents		
Cyclophosphamide	Breast, cervix, head and neck, malignant melanoma, ovary, sarcoma	[27-31]
Melphalan	Breast	[27]
Animetabodies		
Fluorouracil	Bladder, breast, cervix, colon, ovary, pancreas, stomach	[27, 29, 30]
Methotrexate	Breast, cervix, choriocarcinoma, head and neck, ovary, lung	[27, 29-32]
Mitotic inhibitors		
Vinblastine	Breast, malignant melanoma, testis	[27, 29, 33]
Vincristine	Breast, malignant melanoma	[27, 29, 33]
Antibiotics		
Bleomycin	Head and neck, testis	[27, 31]
Dactinomycin	Sarcoma, testis	[27]
Doxorubicin	Bladder, breast, lung, sarcoma	[27, 29]
Other		
Carmustine	Brain, colon, malignant melanoma	[27, 33]
Cisplatin	Bladder, cervix, head and neck, ovary, protate, testis	[30, 31, 34]
Dacarbazine	Malignant melanoma	[33]
Procarbazine	Malignant melanoma	[33]

As an example, in the VAMP combination, vincristine and prednisone having no overlapping toxicity were used at full dose, while the doses of methotrexate and 6-mercaptopurine were reduced to 60% of their maximum tolerated dose as single agents because of their overlapping toxicities.

HODGKIN'S DISEASE

The lessons learned from the results of clinical trials in childhood acute leukemia were first applied to patients with Hodgkin's disease by Dr. Vincent DeVita (Fig. **8.1**) at the National Cancer Institute in 1963. The author recalls vividly, while a medical student, the first course on cancer given by a professor of pathology (pathologists in other medical schools were also often in charge of clinical cancer teaching). The topic was Hodgkin's disease, and the first sentence was: "Hodgkin's disease mostly affects young individuals and is invariably fatal in the advanced stages". A few years later, advanced Hodgkin's disease became curable. A combination of four drugs, mechlorethamine, vincristine (trade name oncovin), methotrexate and prednisone, acronym MOMP, was used initially for a brief period during which modifications in duration of drug administration were studied, based on leukocyte kinetics in experimental animal models and in humans [35, 36].

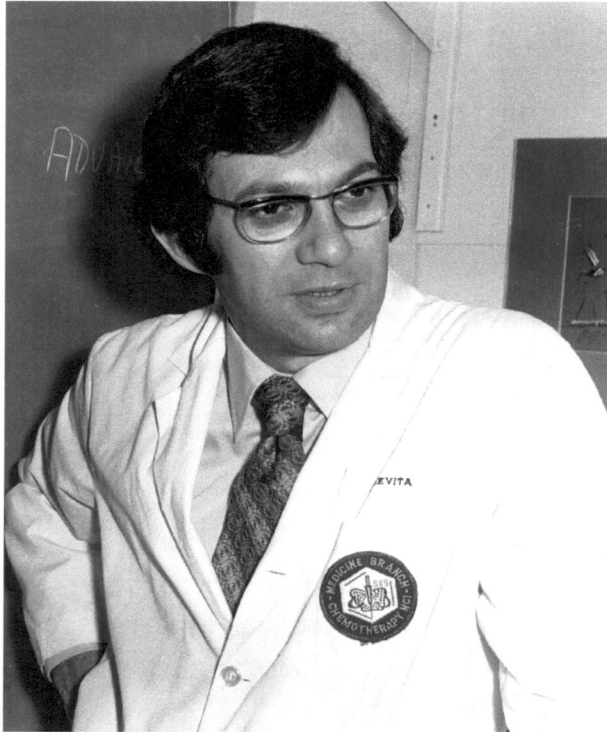

Figure 8.1: Dr. Vincent DeVita. Photograph taken around 1970 kindly provided to the author by Dr. DeVita.

At the same time, reports were being published on a new class of anticancer compounds. "When testing a series of hydrazines for another purpose" some were observed by investigators in Switzerland to have a pronounced antitumor effect in experimental animal systems [37, 38]. One of the compounds, procarbazine, was not only found to induce complete remissions in one-third of the cases of advanced Hodgkin's disease in a Phase II study carried out by Mathé's group in France [26] and by DeVita *et al*. in the United States (reviewed in ref. 36), but also showed no cross-resistance with alkylating agents or vinblastine [26]. Procarbazine was substituted for methotrexate in MOMP which then became known under the acronym MOPP. Of the first 43 cases of advanced Hodgkin's disease treated with MOPP, complete responses were observed in 35 (81%) [39].

In a later publication, DeVita, the principal investigator of the MOPP study had good reasons to state proudly that: "Today, 40 years after the development of combination chemotherapy, Hodgkin's disease patients are cured in approximately 80% of cases, and national mortality rates from the disease have fallen dramatically in the United States [36]".

NON-HODGKIN'S LYMPHOMAS

Non-Hodgkin's lymphomas encompass different histologic subtypes and have different prognoses and responses to therapy. The first study reporting on combination chemotherapy in non-Hodgkin's lymphoma was carried out by two cooperative groups, the ALGB and the ECOG. The remission induction phase compared cyclophosphamide alone to a combination of cyclophosphamide, vincristine and prednisone (acronym COP) resulting in a twofold increase in complete and partial remissions in patients with lymphosarcoma and reticulum cell sarcoma receiving the combination [40]. In another study, the same agents were also given as remission inducers in patients with lymphosarcoma and reticulum cell sarcoma; patients who achieved complete remissions were then randomised to receive maintenance COP or no treatment. The duration of maintained remission was twice as long in patients with lymphosarcoma [41]. Using a different dose-schedule of COP in patients with lymphosarcoma, complete remission occurred in 20 of 35 treated patients; in 89% of these cases, remissions lasted for at least one year after the end of treatment [42]. Survival lasting from one to over seven years after stopping treatment was reported in a study where COP and MOPP were given to 80 patients with advanced non-Hodgkin's lymphoma of various histologic subtypes [43]. The results of these and other early studies using combination chemotherapy were reviewed in 1974 [15]. The following year, complete remissions were achieved in 11 of 27 cases (41%)

of diffuse histiocytic lymphoma (reticulum cell sarcoma). Ten of these remained in complete remission for periods ranging from 26 months to nearly nine years after treatment was discontinued [44].

BURKITT'S LYMPHOMA

Dr. Denis P. Burkitt (1911-1993) was an Irish surgeon and a profoundly religious man who decided to work with people in need. For most of his clinical career he worked at Mulago Hospital in Kampala, Uganda, where in 1957 he saw a young boy with a disfiguring jaw tumor [45]. "His face was massively swollen . . . I had never seen anything like it . . . A few weeks later . . . my attention was attracted by a child with a swollen distorted face sitting on the grass with its mother. I immediately went outside to look at him and, to my surprise recognized precisely the same features as I had observed in the Mulago Hospital ward a few weeks previously. My interest was rivetted immediately. A curiosity can occur once, but two cases indicated more than a curiosity [46]". In 1958, Burkitt (Fig. **8.2**) described the clinical features of 38 cases of "sarcoma" involving the jaws [47]. These tumors were subsequently more precisely characterized as the very rapidly growing lymphoma that now bears his name, Burkitt's lymphoma, a malignancy accounting for about half of all cancers occurring in African children. Most affected children died within 6 months of the onset of symptoms [48]. Treatment with mechlorethamine (nitrogen mustard) or methotrexate led to temporary regressions, and it was concluded that "with the chemotherapeutic compounds at present available, hope for better than very brief remission and perhaps some palliation is dim [48]". However, methotrexate was later shown to induce marked regression of small tumors, whereas cyclophosphamide was noted to produce similar effects even in advanced cases [5]. An addendum to that report stated: "Ten months after this paper was submitted none of the patients who had then survived for a year or more after treatment is known to have died [5]". Impressive results were also obtained with vincristine [16]. In a later study comparing cyclophosphamide alone *versus* a four-drug combination in patients with generalized Burkitt's lymphoma, no significant differences were noted in terms of remission induction, relapse rate or survival; however, two-thirds of the patients who relapsed after receiving a single agent responded to the combination [49].

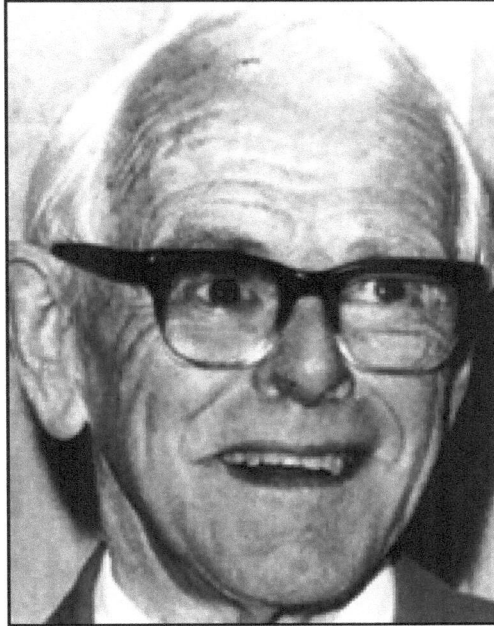

Figure 8.2: Dr. Denis Burkitt. Photograph in: Ferguson A. D.P. Burkitt [obituary] Br Med J 1993; 306:996. Reproduced with permission from BMJ Publishing Group Ltd.

Burkitt's lymphoma became, after choriocarcinoma, the second cancer curable with a single chemotherapeutic drug alone. As Burkitt commented: "I must have been the most ignorant chemotherapist in the world getting the best results—an enviable position [46]".

Burkitt also described the epidemiology of the disease after a ten week "Tumor Safari" of over 10,000 miles across nine African countries [50]. "This form of investigation, touring the African bush in a Ford station wagon that had already seen eight years of service in the Congo, is foreign to accepted concepts of cancer research, but nevertheless proved fruitful [50]". It was noted that the tumors occurred in a distinct geographic area within a belt across Africa where the mean temperature always remained above 15° centigrade and where malaria was holoendemic, that is where essentially all individuals populating the area were infected. These observations provided clues to the factors associated with the etiology of the disease. An interesting aside: it was from biopsy specimens of Burkitt's lymphoma sent by Burkitt that the Epstein-Barr virus was discovered [51].

TESTICULAR CANCER

Testicular cancer although an uncommon tumor in men, was the main cause of cancer death in the 25-to-34 age group before the advent of combination chemotherapy which Li initiated in 1960 [52]. Of 23 patients with metastatic disease treated with a three-drug combination, seven underwent complete or nearly complete responses with improved survival. Li's regimen remained in wide use for over a decade, until clinical investigators at the MD Anderson Hospital in Houston, Texas, reported a 75% response rate in patients treated with vinblastine and bleomycin [53]. The mean survival of complete responders was over two years.

During the investigation of the effect of an electric field on bacterial growth, it was observed that cell division of *Escherichia coli* was inhibited when current passed through platinum electrodes. "Platinum was chosen for the electrode material because of its well-known chemical inertness, and 1,000 c/s (cycles per second) was chosen to eliminate electrolysis effects and electrode polarization. As we will show, both are mistaken ideas which led, *via* serendipity, to the effects described in this communication [54]". It was subsequently found that the growth inhibition was due not to the electric field but to platinum salts released in the medium; one of the compounds, cisplatin, was shown to be the most active against experimental animal tumor systems, and a Phase I study carried out by Holland's group revealed marked activity against advanced testicular cancer [55]. Based on this information, Dr. Lawrence Einhorn (Fig. **8.3**) and colleagues at Indiana University Medical Center in Indianapolis, Indiana, initiated a study in patients with disseminated testicular cancer, adding cisplatin to the vinblastine-bleomycin combination [56]. "Thirty-five of 47 patients (74%) achieved complete remissions; and 29 of these complete remissions remain alive and disease-free at from 6+ to 30+ months". The authors concluded: "We believe this regimen represents a major advance in the management of patients with disseminated testicular cancer [56]".

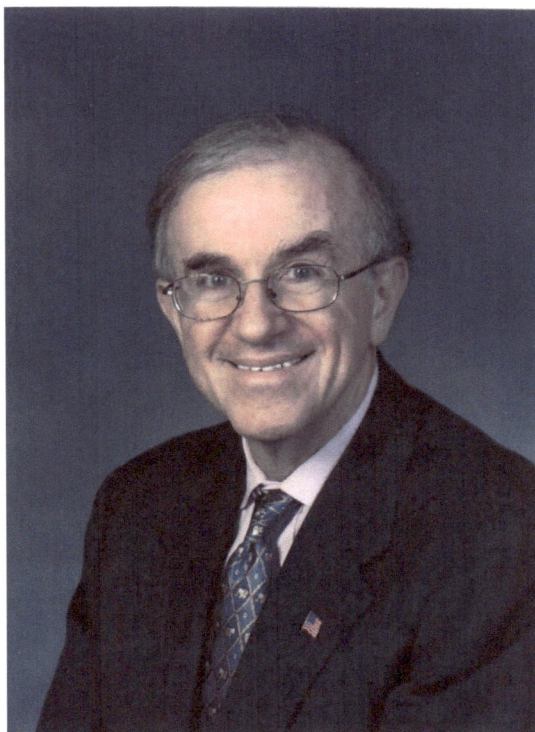

Figure 8.3: Dr. Lawrence Einhorn. Photograph kindly provided to the author by Dr. Einhorn.

In a later publication, Einhorn reported on the outcome of the 47 patients: "The 5 year survival was 64% (30 of 47), and 27 patients (57%) are currently alive and cured of their cancer" and concluded: "There is no question today about the curability of disseminated testicular cancer [57]". The increased survival and decreased mortality rates of testicular cancer in the United States confirmed his assertion [58].

A WORD ON PEDIATRIC CANCER

Fortunately, cancer in the one-to-15 age group is rare with an overall incidence rate of about 133 per million [59]. Excluding acute leukemia, Hodgkin's disease and non-Hodgkin's lymphoma, central nervous system cancers account for about one-third of all other cancers, followed by neuroblastoma (~12%), Wilms'tumor (~10%), rhabdomyosarcoma (~ 6%), osteogenic sarcoma (~ 4%) and Ewing's sarcoma (~ 3%); all other histologic types represent about 28% of cases [59].

Childhood solid tumors used to be largely fatal diseases despite advances in surgery and radiation therapy. In the 1950s, regressions of advanced Wilms's tumor, rhabdomysosarcoma and neuroblastoma were reported with dactinomycin (actinomycin D) [60-62], an antibiotic obtained from bacteria "found in a soil that repeatedly had been fed living bacteria until it had become literally an overflowing cemetery for microorganisms [63]". Subsequently, cyclophosphamide, vincristine and doxorubicin (adriamycin) were noted to have activity as single agents in these and other childhood solid tumors, and methotrexate with leucovorin rescue was shown to induce complete remissions in children with metastatic osteogenic sarcoma [64-69]. Combination chemotherapy and long term maintenance were used, leading to improved survival of pediatric malignancies [70-74].

What may be less appreciated is that chemotherapy was used as the initial form of treatment with the view of rendering inoperable tumors operable [75, 76]. Of great significance, chemotherapy began to be administered in association with radiation therapy in early disease in an attempt to improve survival, and immediately after surgery with a view to preventing metastases [75, 76]. "A long-range program designed to prevent metastases from Wilm's tumor involves the administration of actinomycin D at the time of surgical removal of the primary tumor and local radiotherapy for all patients with Wilm's tumor [75]". The hypothesis was: "In the children with Wilm's tumor who died, the tumor must have metastasized already at the time of discovery of the primary tumor . . . The assumption was made that the clinical agent carried throughout the body by the blood stream might destroy small foci of tumor before solid implantation and further growth could take place [77]". The pioneer pediatric oncologists of the early days were precursors of what later became to be known as combined modality and "adjuvant" chemotherapy, and forerunners of "neoadjuvant" chemotherapy.

The successes in lymphomas, testicular cancer and pediatric cancers were achieved in tumors characterized by rapid cell proliferation [78] and were not paralleled in the common and more slowly growing solid tumors in adults such as lung, breast and colon cancers. However, experimental and clinical analysis of the dynamics of solid tumor growth would provide the insight that led to a revolution in the therapeutic approaches to solid tumors.

REFERENCES

[1]   Galton DA. Myleran in chronic myeloid leukaemia; results of treatment. Lancet 1953; 264:208-13.

[2]   Galton DA, Israels LG, Nabarro JD, Till M. Clinical trials of p-(di-2-chloroethylamino)-phenylbutyric acid (CB 1348) in malignant lymphoma. Br Med J 1955; 2:1172-6.

[3]   Fernbach DJ, Sutow WW, Thurman WG, Vietti TJ. Clinical evalutation of cyclophosphamide. A new agent for the treatment of children with acute leukemia. JAMA 1962; 182:30-7.

[4]   Matthias JQ, Misiewicz JJ, Scott RB. Cycloposphamide in Hodgkin's disease and related disorders. Br Med J 1960; 2:1837-40.

[5]   Burkitt D, Hutt MSR, Wright DH. The African lymphoma. Preliminary observations on response to therapy. Cancer 1965; 18:399-410.

[6]   Eckhardt S, Sellei C, Horvath IP, Institorisz L. Effect of 1, 6-dibromo- 1, 6-dideoxy-D-mannitol on chronic granulocytic leukemia. Cancer Chemother Rep 1963; 33:57-61.

[7]   Waldenström J. Melphalan therapy in myelomatosis. Br Med J 1964; 1:859-65.

[8]   Goodman LS, Wintrobe MM, Dameshek W, Goodman MJ, Gilman A, McLennan MT. Nitrogen mustard therapy; use of methyl-bis (beta-chloroethyl) amine hydrochloride and tris (beta-chloroethyl) amine hydrochloride for Hodgkin's disease, lymphosarcoma, leukemia and certain allied and miscellaneous disorders. JAMA 1946; 132:126-32.

[9]   Ellison RR, Holland JF, Weil M, *et al.* Arabinosyl cytosine: a useful agent in the treatment of acute leukemia in adults. Blood 1968; 32:507-23.

[10]   Traggis DG, Dohlwitz A, Das L, Jaffe N, Moloney WC, Hall TC. Cytosine arabinoside in acute leukemia of childhood. Cancer 1971; 28:815-8.

[11]   Holland JF, Frei E III. Cancer Medicine. Philadelphia, Lea and Febiger, 1973; pp. 618-21.

[12]   Oettgen HF, Burkitt D, Burchenal JH. Malignant lymphoma involving the jaw in African children: treatment with methotrexate. Cancer 1963; 16:616-23.

[13]   Johnson IS, Armstrong JG, Gorman M, Burnett JP Jr. The vinca alkaloids: a new class of oncolytic agents. Cancer Res 1963; 23:1390-427.

[14]   Carter SK, Livingston RB. Single-agent therapy for Hodgkin's disease. Arch Intern Med 1973; 131:377-87.

[15]   Bonadonna G, Monfardini S. Chemotherapy of non-Hodgkin's lymphomas. Cancer Treat Rev 1974; 1:167-81.

[16]   Burkitt D. African lymphoma. Observations on response to vincristine sulphate therapy. Cancer 1966; 19:1131-7.

[17]   Blum RH, Carter SK, Agre K. A clinical review of bleomycin—a new antineoplastic agent. Cancer 1973; 31:903-14.

[18]   Jacquillat C, Boiron M, Weil M, Tanzer J, Najean Y, Bernard J. Rubidomycin. A new agent active in the treatment of acute lymphoblastic leukaemia. Lancet 1966; 2:27-8.

[19]   Bernard J. Acute leukemia treatment. Cancer Res 1967; 27:2565-9.

[20]   Tan C, Tasaka H, Yu KP, Murphy ML, Karnofsky DA. Daunomycin, an antitumor antibiotic, in the treatment of neoplastic disease. Clinical evaluation with special reference to childhood leukemia. Cancer 1967; 20:333-53.

[21]   Blum RH, Carter SK. Adriamycin. A new anticancer drug with significant clinical activity. Ann Int Med 1974; 80:249-59.

[22]   Whitecar JP Jr, Bodey GP, Harris JE, Freireich EJ. L-Asparaginase. N Engl J Med 1970; 282:732-4.

[23]   Carter SK, Schabel FM, Broder LE, Johnston TP. 1, 3-bis (2-chloroethyl)-1-nitrosourea (BCNU) and other nitrosoureas in cancer treatment— a review. Adv Cancer Res 1972; 16:273-332.

[24]   Frei E 3rd, Luce JK, Talley RW, Vaitkevicius VK, Wilson HE. 5-(3,3-dimethyl-1-triazeno) imidazole-4-carboxamide (NSC-45388) in the treatment of lymphoma. Cancer Chemother Rep 1972; 56:667-70.

[25]   Kennedy BJ, Yarbro JW. Metabolic and therapeutic effects of hydroxyurea in chronic myeloid leukemia. JAMA 1966; 195:1038-43.

[26]   Mathé G, Schweisguth O, Schneider M, *et al.* Mehtyl-hydrazine in treatment of Hodgkin's disease and various forms of haematosarcoma and leukaemia. Lancet 1963; 2:1077-80.

[27]   Carter SK, Soper WT. Integration of chemotherapy into combined modality treatment of solid tumors. 1. The overall strategy. Cancer Treat Rev 1974; 1:1-13.

[28]   Carter SK, Livingston RB. Cyclophosphamide in solid tumors. Cancer Treat Rev 1975; 2:295-322.

[29]   Carbone PP, Bauer M, Band P, Tormey D. Chemotherapy of disseminated breast cancer. Current status and prospects. Cancer 1977; 39 (6 Suppl):2916-22.

[30]   Young RC, Hubbard SP, DeVita VT. The chemotherapy of ovarian carcinoma. Cancer Treat Rev 1974; 1:99-110.

[31]   Bertino JR, Boston B, Capizzi RL. The role of chemotherapy in the management of cancer of the head and neck: a review. Cancer 1975; 36:752-8.

[32]   Li MC, Hertz B, Spencer DB. Effect of methotrexate therapy upon choriocarcinoma and chorioadenoma. Proc Soc Exp Biol Med 1956; 93:361-66.

[33]   Luce JK. Chemotherapy of malignant melanoma. Cancer 1972; 30:1604-15.

[34]   Prestayko AW, D'Aoust JC, Issell BF, Crooke ST. Cisplatin (*cis*-diamminedichloroplatinum II). Cancer Treat Rev 1979; 6:17-39.

[35]   Frei E III. Combination cancer therapy: Presidential address. Cancer Res 1972; 32:2593-607.

[36]   DeVita VT Jr. A selective history of the therapy of Hodgkin's disease. Brit J Haematol 2003; 122:718-27.

[37]   Zeller P, Gutmann H, Hegedüs B, Kaiser A, Langemann A, Müller M. Methylhydrazine derivatives, a new class of cytotoxic agents. Experientia 1963; 19:129.

[38]   Bollag W, Grunberg E. Tumor inhibitory effects of a new class of cytotoxic agents: methylhydrazine derivatives. Experientia 1963; 19:130-1.

[39]   DeVita VT Jr, Serpick AA, Carbone PP. Combination chemotherapy in the treatment of advanced Hodgkin's disease. Ann Intern Med 1970; 73:881-95.

[40]   Hoogstraten B, Owens AH, Lenhard RE, *et al.* Combination chemotherapy in lymphosarcoma and reticulum cell sarcoma. Blood 1969; 33:370-8.

[41]   Luce JK, Gamble JF, Wilson HE, *et al.* Combined cyclophosphamide, vincristine, and prednisone therapy of malignant lymphoma. Cancer 1971; 28:306-17.

[42]   Bagley CM Jr, DeVita VT Jr, Berard CW, Canellos GP. Advanced lymphosarcoma: intensive cyclical combination chemotherapy with cyclophosphamide, vinciristine and prednisone. Ann Intern Med 1972; 76:227-234.

[43]   Schein PS, Chabner BA, Canellos GP, Young RC, Berard C, DeVita VT. Potential for prolonged disease-free survival following combination chemotherapy of non-Hodgkin's lymphoma. Blood 1974; 43:181-9.

[44]   DeVita VT Jr, Chabner B, Hubbard SP, Canellos GP, Schein P, Young RC. Advanced diffuse histiocytic lymphoma, a potentially curable disease: results with combination chemotherapy. Lancet 1975; 1:248-50.

[45]   Coakley D. Denis Burkitt and his contribution to haematology/oncology. Br J Haematol 2006; 135:17–25.

[46]   Burkitt DP. The discovery of Burkitt's lymphoma. Cancer 1983; 51:1777-86.

[47]   Burkitt D. A sarcoma involving the jaws in African children. Br J Surg 1958; 46:218-23.

[48]   Burkitt D, O'Conor GT. Malignant lymphoma in African children. I. A clinical syndrome. Cancer 1961; 14:258-69.

[49]   Ziegler JL, Bluming AZ, Magrath IT, Carbone PP. Intensive chemotherapy in patients with generalized Burkitt's lymphoma. Int J Cancer 1972; 10:254-61.

[50]   Burkitt D. A "Tumour Safari" in East and Central Africa. Br J Cancer 1962; 16:379-86.

[51]   Epstein MA, Achong BG, Barr YM. Virus particles in cultured lymphoblasts from Burkitt's lymphoma. Lancet 1964; 1:702-3.

[52]   Li MC, Whitmore WF Jr, Golbey R, Grabstald H. Effects of combined drug therapy on metastatic cancer of the testis. JAMA 1960; 174:1291-9.

[53]   Samuels ML, Holoye PY, Johnson DE. Bleomycin combination chemotherapy in the management of testicular neoplasia. Cancer 1975; 36:318-26.

[54]   Rosenberg B, Van Camp L, Krigas T. Inhibition of cell division in *Escherichia coli* by electrolysis products from a platinum electrode. Nature 1965; 205:698-9.

[55]   Higby DJ, Wallace HJ Jr, Albert DJ, Holland JF. Diaminodichloroplatinum: a phase I study showing responses in testicular and other tumors. Cancer 1974; 33:1219-25.

[56]   Einhorn LH, Donohue J. *Cis*-diamminedichloroplatinum, vinblastine, and bleomycin combination chemotherapy in disseminated testicular cancer. Ann Intern Med 1977; 87:293-8.

[57]   Einhorn LH. Testicular cancer as a model for a curable neoplasm: the Richard and Hinda Rosenthal Foundation Award Lecture. Cancer Res 1981; 41:3275-80.

[58]   Li FP, Connelly RR, Myers M. Improved survival rates among testis cancer patients in the United States. JAMA 1982; 247:825-6.

[59]   Gurney JG, Severson RK, Davis S, Robison LL. Incidence of cancer in children in the United States. Sex-, race-, and 1-year age-specific rates by histologic type. Cancer 1995; 75:2186-95.

[60]   Farber S, Pinkel D, Sears EM, Toch R. Advances in chemotherapy of cancer in man. Adv Cancer Res 1956; 4:1-71.

[61]   Tan CTC, Dargeon HW, Burchenal JH. The effect of actinomycin D on cancer in childhood. Pediatrics 1959; 24:544-61.

[62]   Pinkel D. Actinomycin D in childhood cancer; a preliminary report. Pediatrics 1959; 23:342-7.

[63]   Woodruff HB, Waksman SA. The actinomycins and their importance in the treatment of tumors in animals and man. Historical background. Ann NY Acad Sci 1960; 89:287-98.

[64]   Pinkel D. Cyclophosphamide in children with cancer. Cancer 1962; 15:42-9.

[65]   Pinkel D, Pickren J. Rhabomyosarcoma in children. JAMA 1961; 175:293-8.

[66]   Selawry OS, Hananian J. Vincristine treatment of cancer in children. JAMA 1963; 183:741-6.

[67]   James DH Jr, George P. Vincristine in children with malignant solid tumors. J Pediatr 1964; 64:534-41.

[68]   Tan C, Etcubanas E, Wollner N, *et al*. Adriamycin--an antitumor antibiotic in the treatment of neoplastic diseases. Cancer 1973; 32:9-17.

[69]   Jaffe N, Paed D. Recent advances in the chemotherapy of metastatic osteogenic sarcoma. Cancer 1972; 30:1627-31.

[70]   Hustu HO, Holton C, James D Jr, Pinkel D. Treatment of Ewing's sarcoma with concurrent radiotherapy and chemotherapy. J Pediatr 1968; 73:249-51.

[71]   Pinkel D, Pratt C, Holton C, James D Jr, Wrenn E Jr, Hustu HO. Survival of children with neuroblastoma treated with combination chemotherapy. J Pediatr 1968; 73:928-31.

[72]   Pratt CB. Response of childhood rhabdomyosarcoma to combination chemotherapy. J Pediatr 1969; 74:791-4.

[73]   Wolff JA, Krivit W, Newton WA Jr, D'Angio GJ. Single *versus* multiple dose dactinomycin therapy of Wilms's tumor. A controlled co-operative study conducted by the Children's Cancer Study Group A (formerly Acute Leukemia Co-operative Chemotherapy Group A). N Engl J Med 1968; 279:290-4.

[74]   Murphy ML. Curability of cancer in children. Cancer 1968; 22:779-84.

[75]   Farber S, D'Angio G, Evans A, Mitus A. Clinical studies of actinomycin D with special reference to Wilm's tumor in children. Ann NY Acad Sci 1960; 89:421-5.

[76]   James DH Jr, George P, Hustu O, *et al*. Chemotherapy of localized inoperable malignant tumors of children. Preliminary report. JAMA 1964; 189:636-8.

[77]   Farber S. Chemotherapy in the treatment of leukemia and Wilms' tumor. JAMA 1966; 198:826-36.

[78]   Shackney SE, McCormack GW, Cuchural GJ Jr. Growth rate patterns of solid tumors and their relation to responsiveness to therapy: an analytical review. Ann Int Med 1978; 89:107-21.

"Clinical diagnosis is a late event in the natural history of neoplastic growth".
Dr. Mordechai Schwartz.

CHAPTER 9

Tumor Growth

Pierre R. Band[*]

Department of Medicine, McGill University, Montreal, Canada

Abstract: The growth rates of solid tumors in experimental animals and in humans were found to be exponential during their observable lifetime. It was concluded that cancer develops over a long clinically undetectable phase, during which the probability of occurrence of metastases is high. Solid tumors became viewed as frequently disseminated at the time of clinical diagnosis, thus requiring a systemic therapeutic approach in addition to the traditional loco-regional approaches offered by surgery or radiation therapy. However, studies in experimental animal models in which tumor growth can be measured over a wide range of doubling times have shown that solid tumor growth rates best fit a Gompertz function, in which the tumor doubling times continuously increase with increasing tumor size. Subsequent studies of the dynamics of tumor growth revealed that tumors are composed of proliferative and non-proliferative compartments, the latter consisting of cells that are able to proliferate again and cells lacking this capacity. In addition to therapeutic implications drawn from the Gompertz and cell-compartment models, experimental tumors characterized by a Gompertzian growth were added to the *in vivo* systems used to screen for drug activity.

Keywords: Tumor growth rate, exponential, Gompertzian, screening systems.

THE EXPERIMENTAL AND CLINICAL GROWTH RATES OF TUMORS ARE EXPONENTIAL DURING THEIR VISIBLE LIFE

In 1935, a British pathologist, Dr. J. Cecil Mottram (1880-1945) published results on the growth rate of carcinogen-induced skin epitheliomas in mice [1]. By plotting the logarithms of tumor areas against time, he observed that the growth rate was exponential during the tumor's visible life and inferred that "if tar epitheliomas take origin from a single cell they must show a long latent period

*Address correspondence to Pierre R. Band: Faculty of Medicine, McGill University, Montreal, Quebec H3G 1Y6, Canada; E-mail: pierre.band@gmail.com

between their origin and their first appearance on the skin as visible warts [1]". He estimated the approximate area of a single cell and calculated the time of inception of the tumor by extrapolating the growth curve backward to the area of a single cell. His conclusion was: "it takes long periods of time . . . for single cells to grow to visible warts [1]". Furthermore, he drew attention to tumour doubling and estimated the volume of 1,000,000 cells to be approximately one cubic millimetre. Mottram could not predict the future of his observations, which heralded the very foundation of medical oncology, namely the concept of cancer as a systemic disease. Mottram is also remembered for his classical work on carcinogenesis: "He shewed that benzpyrene could produce tumours in mice by a single application of this substance on the skin, but only when it was associated with croton oil; the function of the latter is to increase the cellular activity of the cell [2]".

Two decades later, Collins *et al.* from the Department of Radiology at Baylor University College of Medicine in Houston, Texas, were the first to study the growth rate of human cancer [3]. "If the growth rate of the hypothetical tumor were constant it could be described in terms of 'doubling time'. . . According to this hypothesis, a single cancer cell 10μ in diameter will grow to a nodule 1mm . . . A 1 cm nodule, a likely size for early diagnosis, would be achieved in 30 doublings. A further ten doublings will produce approximately one kilogram of cancer tissue . . . Thus the total maximum duration of cancer is of the order of time required for 40 doublings in volume and half of this occurs in a period of undetected growth prior to the earliest possible sign of symptom [3]". These authors followed the volumetric growth of pulmonary metastases from various primary sites at known time intervals in 24 patients. When the tumor volumes were plotted on a semilogarithmic scale, the growth curve became a straight line reflecting the exponential growth rate that was found to be specific for individual tumors. Tumor growth was clearly described in terms of doubling times, which were classified into rapid (less than 25 days), intermediate (25 to 74 days) and slow growing (75 days and over). By projecting the slope of the growth curves backward to the volume of one cell, the time when cancer originated was estimated and the following conclusions provided:

"Evidence is added that the duration of cancer before diagnosis may be very long".

"The long duration of the period of undetected growth of cancer . . . offers an explanation for the failure of early diagnosis to influence cure, survival, or mortality rates".

"The failures of treatment are largely due to undetected metastases present at the time of treatment".

"Therapeutic effort must be directed to the period of undetected growth if behavior and outcome are to be altered beyond the level of current achievement [3]".

This seminal paper shattered the concepts of early diagnosis and the misleading notion of five-year cure statistics. More importantly, it radically changed the concept of cancer which, from then on became largely viewed as a systemic disease at the time of clinical diagnosis.

To illustrate, when a tumor cell divides, it gives rise to two daughter cells. Thus, after the first doubling, two cells are produced, four after the second, and eight after the third doubling. After a hypothetical 3.3 doublings there will be 10 cells, so after 9.9 or about 10 doublings the number of cells in the population will be 1,000. It will be 1 million after 20, 1 billion after 30 and 1 trillion after 40 doublings. It is difficult to relate to these astronomical numbers unless a measure can be associated with them (Table **9.1**).

Table 9.1: Tumor diameter and weight by cell doubling and cell number.

Doubling	Cells	Diameter (cm)	Weight
10	10^3	0.01	1 µg
20	10^6	0.1	1 mg
30	10^9	1.0	1 g
40	10^{12}	10.0	1 kg

A tumor containing 1 million cells has an approximate diameter of 0.1 cm, or 1 mm weighs about 1 mg and can't be detected with current techniques. It can, however, be detected by cytology, which explains the success of the Pap test in early detection of cancer of the cervix. In general, the clinical detection of a solid tumor occurs around the 30th doubling, when the tumor diameter is about 1 cm and the cell number around 1 billion, although smaller tumors may be detected at a lesser diameter, for instance with mammography. With 10 more doublings, the tumor reaches a diameter of about 10 centimeters and weighs 1 kilogram, the limit of tolerance of the human host; at around the 40th doubling, death will occur. These relationships are more strikingly apparent on a graph (Fig. **9.1**). Thus, when a tumor is diagnosed two-thirds of its life span has taken place during a long clinically silent period, and after 10 additional doublings death supervenes. During this long pre-clinical period, metastases have a high probability of formation. Holland called these considerations the catechism of medical oncologists. Hence, with the exception of early stage tumors that are potentially curable by surgery or radiation therapy, solid tumors became viewed as frequently disseminated at the time of clinical diagnosis, thus requiring a systemic therapeutic approach beyond the loco-regional approaches offered by surgery or radiation therapy.

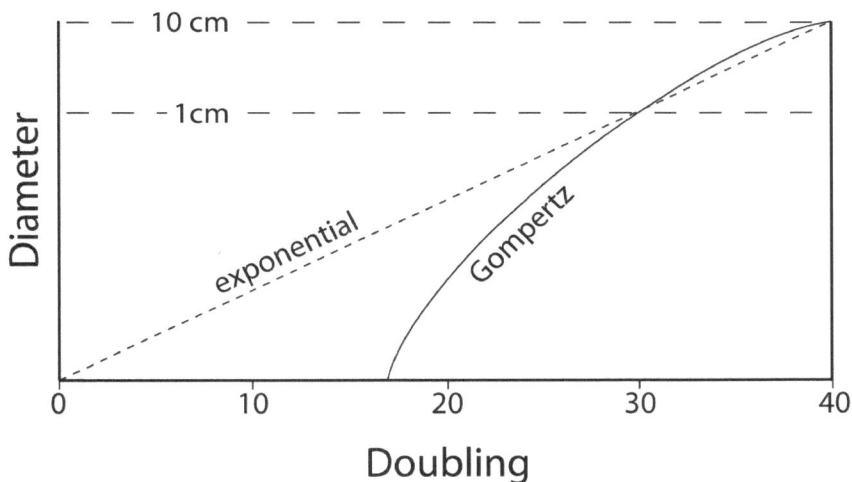

Figure 9.1: Backward extrapolation of exponential and Gompertzian tumor growth rates.

An example of exponential tumor growth, taken from chest X-rays of a patient with liposarcoma who was under the care of the author, is shown in Figs. **9.2** and **9.3**. Because of the intermediate growth rate (doubling time = 41 days) and the possibility of life-threatening metastases, the single lesion was removed.

Several building blocks were added to this solid foundation. First, tumor growth was proposed as a means of testing the effect of chemotherapeutic agents: "Direct observation of changes in tumor mass seems the most reliable method of determining the effect of antitumor agents [4]".

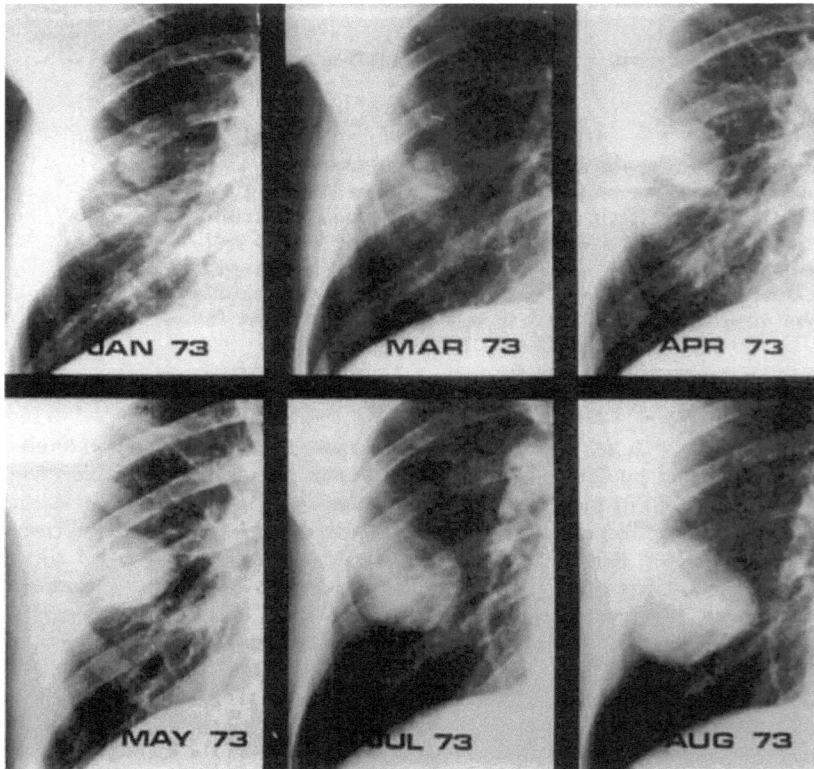

Figure 9.2: Serial roentgenograms of a measurable spherical pulmonary metastasis in an untreated patient with liposarcoma. The visual impression is that the tumor is growing regularly. Fig. **1** in: Band PR, Kocandrle C. Growth rate of pulmonary metastases in human sarcomas. Cancer 1975; 36:471-4, reference 13. Reproduced with permission from John Wiley and Sons.

Second, criteria for patient selection, technique of measurement, and selection of lesion were proposed without, however, suggesting criteria for response based on therapeutically induced tumor growth variation [4]. Third, the mathematical basis for evaluation of exponential tumor growth rates was described, the general validity of the exponential growth rate confirmed, and the long pre-clinical "iceberg" phase of tumor growth emphasized [5]. In a study of untreated pulmonary metastases, a statistical correlation between the most rapidly growing metastases and survival was observed, as well as a variation in growth rate for different metastases in the same patient [6].

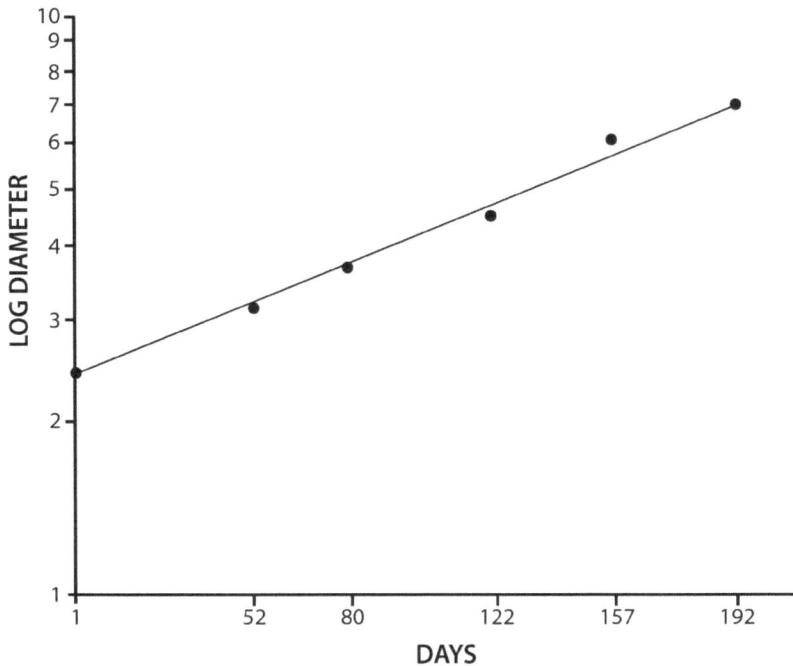

Figure 9.3: Semilogarithmic plot of the lesions measured in Fig. **9.2**.

A study of patients who received palliative radiation therapy to pulmonary metastases of known pretreatment growth rate added the new and very important observation that after treatment, the growth of solid tumors resumed at the original exponential rate: "It follows, that the development of a tumor is set back by irradiation, by a time interval equal to the time necessary to again reach the original volume. This means that a dose of radiation which gives but unsatisfactory reduction in the diameter of a slowly growing tumour still can effect a considerable prolongation of survival time [7]". Finnish investigators observed the same effect with chemotherapy and also concluded: "If the growth rate is the same after treatment as before, one finds that in slow growing tumours a certain decrease in volume caused by treatment results in a longer 'remission' or delay than in rapidly growing tumours experiencing the same decrease [8]". Deviation from the exponential growth rate was found to be uncommon, occurring mainly when the tumor reached a very large size or in relation to hormonal influence, for instance the decline in breast cancer growth rate around menopause [5, 7].

CHEMOTHERAPEUTIC IMPLICATIONS OF EXPONENTIAL TUMOR GROWTH

The implications for chemotherapy of exponential tumor growth were to be fully exploited by Doctors Lucien Israël (Fig. **9.4**) and Philippe Chahinian at the *Centre Hospitalier Universitaire Cochin* in Paris. Israël's specialty was pulmonary medicine; after tuberculosis was cured with triple therapy, patients with lung cancer replaced tuberculosis cases in hospital wards. Israël switched his interest from pulmonary infectious diseases to lung cancer and was among the pioneers of solid tumor combination chemotherapy. Reflecting that tuberculosis could rarely be cured with one drug due to the emergence of drug resistance but cure became possible with three agents, Israël applied the same principle to the treatment of lung cancer [9, 10].

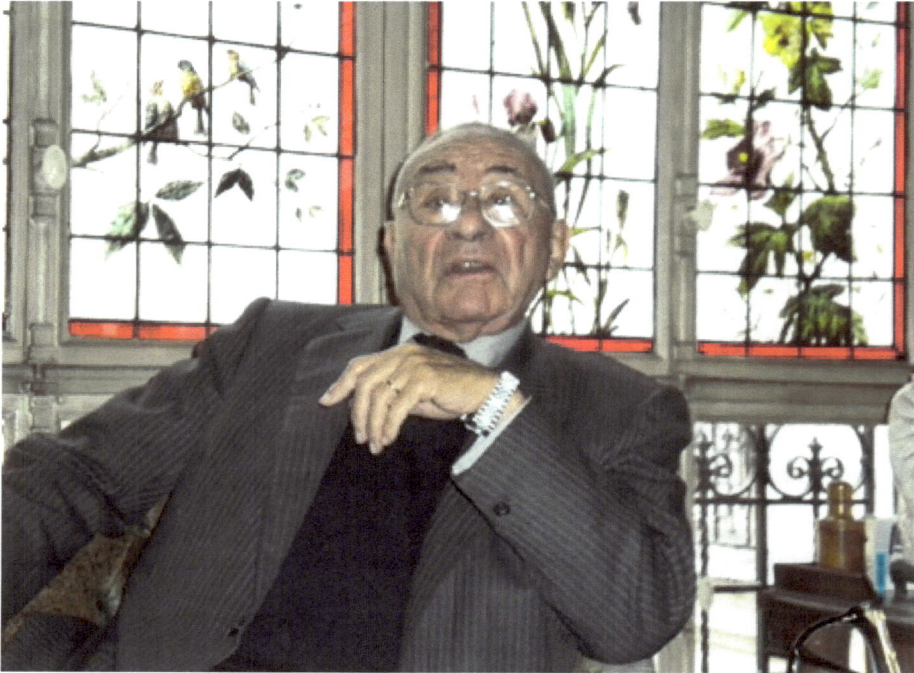

Figure 9.4: Dr. Lucien Israël. Photo taken by the author; Paris, September 2009. Author's collection.

His prominent work in approaches to testing clinical activity of new anticancer agents, inferred from a mathematical model of tumor growth, has largely been overlooked. First, based on arithmetic and trigonometric considerations, Chahinian and Israël developed a mathematical model describing the relationship between the slopes of the spontaneous pre-treatment and the therapeutically induced tumor doubling times. A graphic representation of this model made it possible to calculate the "survival gain ", that is the gain in survival attributable to different therapeutic responses; this could readily be evaluated as the slope of the tumor growth rate becomes parallel to the spontaneous pre-therapeutic slope when drug resistance supervenes [7, 8]. The ratio of the survival gain (SG) to the treatment duration (T), SG/T, made it possible to evaluate the effectiveness of a given treatment quantitatively in cases of different spontaneous pre-therapeutic doubling times. If SG/T = 0, the doubling time is not modified by treatment and the tumor keeps growing at the same rate; if SG/T < 1, the doubling time is lengthened; the tumor continues to grow, but at a reduced rate; if SG/T = 1, the doubling time is abolished and the tumor stops growing; if SG/T > 1, the doubling time becomes negative; the tumor decreases in volume [11]. These relationships are illustrated in Fig. **9.5**.

In a follow-up publication, the authors established the validity of the model in the clinical setting [12]. Specifically, they confirmed that the same treatment of lung cancers of various doubling times led to different SG/T results, including no effect as well as lengthening, arrest and decrease in tumor doubling time. They stated: "The evaluation of chemotherapeutic treatment relies generally . . . on approximative measurement of the shrinkage of the tumor. When considering the growth curves of measurable tumors prior to and during the treatment one can, however, easily reach the conclusion that these parameters are not significative [12]". The authors rightly concluded that "the screening tests overlook drugs which, although not producing a volume reduction, are capable of multiplying by a factor of 5 the time of spontaneous doubling, a result which can hardly be ignored". The usefulness of the model to establish the optimum dose-schedule of drugs in tumors with various doubling times has also been suggested [13].

It should be pointed out that tumor growth rates were, at the time, mostly measured from chest X-rays. With the availability of new radiological techniques and equipment, tumor volumes may readily be obtained, which not only facilitates measurements but substantially boosts the potential for assessing the effects of treatment on the growth rate of tumors at various anatomical sites.

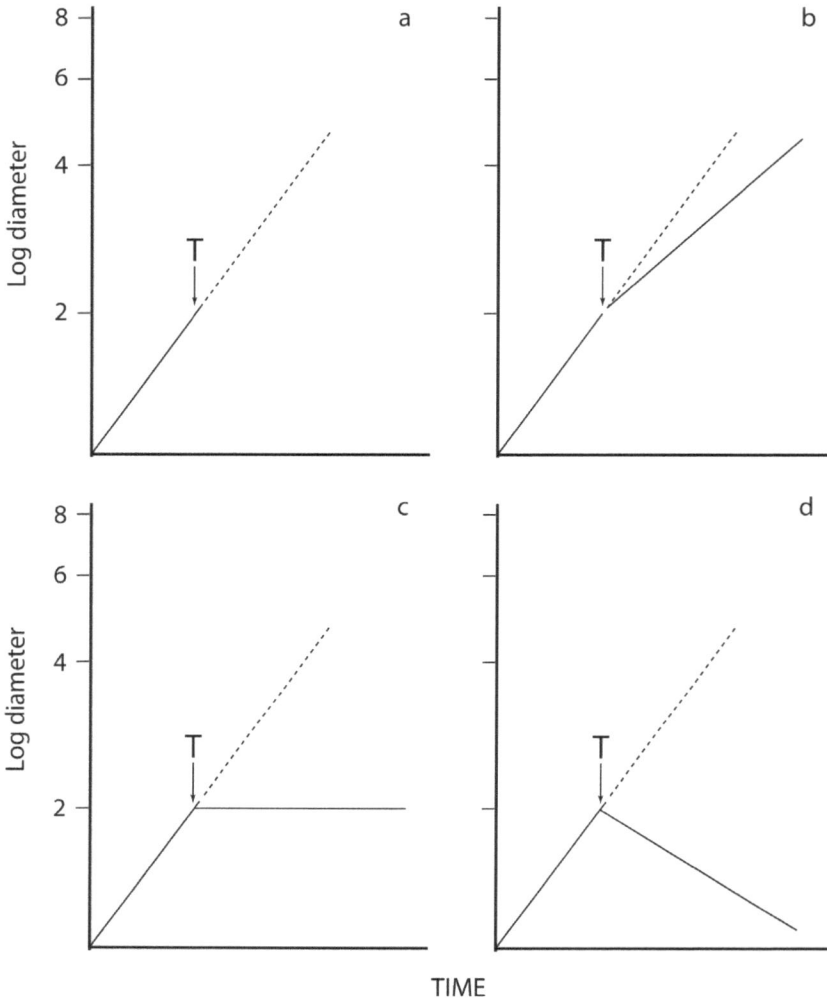

Figure 9.5: Effect of treatment (T) on tumor growth rate; panel a: no effect, tumor grows at pre-therapy rate; panel b: tumor growth rate prolonged; panel c: tumor growth rate arrested; panel d: tumor regression.

FOR MOST EXPERIMENTAL AND CLINICAL TUMORS, GROWTH RATES ARE NOT EXPONENTIAL THROUGHOUT THEIR LIFESPAN

The exponential growth rate of human solid tumors, derived from measurements over a few doublings, was found to be generally valid during the clinical phase of tumor growth. However, studies in experimental animal models for which tumor growth can be measured over a wider range of doubling times have shown that the growth rates of solid tumors best fit a Gompertz function, named after the British mathematician Benjamin Gompertz (1779-1865), in which tumor doubling time continuously increases with increasing tumor size [14]. "When we consider those tumors whose growth has been followed over a sufficiently extensive range (100 to 1000-fold range of growth or more), we find that nearly all such tumors grow more and more slowly as the tumor gets larger . . . Tumor cells proliferate by a modified exponential process in which successive doublings occur at increasingly longer intervals [14]". Notwithstanding, some of the inferences emanating from the exponential model remain unaltered: 1) A large proportion of a tumor lifespan occurs during a clinically silent period; 2) Clinical assessment of the effects of chemotherapeutic drugs using the exponential model is not invalid: over a few doublings, when tumors may be visualized, the exponential and Gompertz curves overlap (Fig. **9.1**). On the other hand, the exponential model overestimates the time of tumor inception (Fig. **9.1**). Of added importance, the two mathematical models have certain therapeutic consequences in common. The therapeutic implications of the first order kinetics concept were derived from the L1210 leukemia exponential model of tumor growth. Similarly, the Gompertz model led to therapeutic inferences that will be addressed in a later chapter.

UNRAVELLING THE DYNAMICS OF TUMOR GROWTH

The L1210 experimental model from which several important principles of chemotherapy were derived is not representative of all experimental and human solid tumors. In other words, cancer in general does not consist of one compartment of proliferating cells. Using cell labeling and autoradiography, it was observed that the proportion of labeled cells with mitotic figures exceeded that of all labeled cells in the tumor population. This gave rise to the hypothesis: "The possibility exists that, like the normal tissues from whence they arose, various tumors are mixtures of proliferating and non-proliferating cells [15]". Experimental evidence for a two-compartment model of solid tumors made up of growing and non-growing cells was first provided by Dr. Mortimer L. Mendelsohn. He proposed the term "growth fraction" for this phenomenon, defining it as the ratio of proliferating cells to the total tumor cell population [15]. He also showed that the mean growth fraction of multiple autotransplants of a primary breast cancer in mice was about 60% [16].

Cell loss from tumors is another process that explains the discrepancy between the potential doubling time computed from the average cell cycle time of the tumor population and the actual tumor doubling time. Described in 1968 by Dr. G. Gordon Steel from the Institute of Cancer Research in Belmont, England, cell loss "expresses the loss of growth potential by the tumour [17]". It is mainly due to cell death, but also to metastases and exfoliation. Cell loss was defined as "the rate of loss of cells as a fraction of the rate at which cells are being added to the tumour volume by mitosis [17]". A high rate of cell loss has been inferred from kinetic studies of experimental and human cancers [17-20]. Experimental evidence suggested that cell loss increases and the growth fraction decreases as tumors grow larger [17, 19, 21]. Thus, both increasing cell loss and a decreasing growth fraction were considered to be major factors underlying Gompertzian tumor growth kinetics.

The two-compartment model of tumor growth, proliferative and non-proliferative, was further refined by separating the non-proliferating compartment into three cellular components: cells that are permanently non-proliferating; non-proliferating cells that retain the capacity to re-enter the proliferative compartment upon an appropriate stimulus (G_0 cells); and cell loss [22].

The description of Gompertzian tumor growth kinetics led to therapeutic and other considerations. It has been aptly argued that only clonogenic (stem) proliferating and G_0 cells need to be considered for therapeutic purposes [22, 23]; as well, the use of cell-cycle specific and nonspecific agents was suggested in order to eradicate both cellular components [21]. Another important implication was the addition to the experimental animal screening systems of tumor models, such as the B16 melanoma and the Lewis lung transplantable mouse tumors, which had Gompertzian kinetics more in keeping with the growth characteristics of human solid tumors than the L1210 leukemia model [24-26].

REFERENCES

[1]   Mottram JC. On the origin of tar tumours in mice, whether from single cells or many cells. J Path Bact 1935; 40:407-14.
[2]   Russ S. The scientific work of Dr JC Mottram (1880-1945). Brit J Radiol 1946; 19:347-8.
[3]   Collins VP, Loeffler RK, Tivey H. Observations on growth rates of human tumors. Am J Roentgenol Radium Ther Nucl Med 1956; 76:988-1000.
[4]   Brindley CO, Markoff E, Schneiderman MA. Direct observation of lesion size and number as a method of following the growth of human tumors. Cancer 1959; 12:139-46.
[5]   Schwartz M. A biomathematical approach to clinical tumor growth. Cancer 1961; 14:1272-94.

[6]   Spratt JS Jr, Spratt TL. Rates of growth of pulmonary metastases and host survival. Ann Surg 1964; 159:161-71.

[7]   Breur K. Growth rate and radiosensitivity of human tumours. II. Radiosensitivity of human tumors. Eur J Cancer 1966; 2:173-88.

[8]   Brenner MW, Holsti LR, Perttala Y. The study by graphical analsis of the growth of human tumours and metastases of the lung. Br J Cancer 1967; 21:1-13.

[9]   Israël L, Sors C, Bernard E. Prolonged polychemotherapy of inoperable bronchopulmonary cancers. À propos of 165 cases. Sem Hop 1966; 42:1825-9.

[10]   Israël L. Anticancer polychemotherapy of human tumors. Theoretical and practical problems. Poumon Coeur. 1968; 24:15-9.

[11]   Chahinian P, Israël L. Survival gain and volume gain. Mathematical tools in evaluating treatments. Eur J Cancer 1969; 5:625-9.

[12]   Israel L, Chahinian P. Evaluation of the survival gain in 22 measurable lung tumors treated with chemotherapy. An approach towards quantitative evaluation of cancer treatments in man. Eur J Cancer 1969; 5:631-7.

[13]   Band PR, Kocandrle C. Growth rate of pulmonary metastases in human sarcomas. Cancer 1975; 36:471-4.

[14]   Laird AK. Dynamics of tumor growth. Br J Cancer 1964; 13:490-502.

[15]   Mendelsohn ML. The growth fraction: a new concept applied to tumors. Science 1960; 132:1496.

[16]   Mendelsohn ML. Autoradiographic analysis of cell proliferation in spontaneous breast cancer of C3H mouse. III. The growth fraction. JNatl Cancer Inst 1962; 28:1015-29.

[17]   Steel GG. Cell loss from experimental tumours. Cell Tissue Kinet 1968; 1:193-207.

[18]   Steel GG. Cell loss as a factor in the growth rate of human tumours. Eur J Cancer 1967; 3:381-7.

[19]   Frindel E, Malaise EP, Alpen E, Tubiana M. Kinetics of cell proliferation of an experimental tumor. Cancer Res 1967; 27:1122-31.

[20]   Frindel E, Malaise E, Tubiana M. Cell proliferation kinetics in five human solid tumors. Cancer 1968; 22:611-20.

[21]   Schabel FM Jr. The use of tumor growth kinetics in planning "curative" chemotherapy of advanced solid tumors. Cancer Res 1969; 29:2384-9.

[22]   Mendelsohn ML. Cell cycle kinetics and mitotically linked chemotherapy. Cancer Res 1969; 29:2390-3.

[23]   Skipper HE. Kinetics of mammary tumor cell growth and implications for therapy. Cancer 1971; 28:1479-99.

[24]   Johnson RK, Goldin A. The clinical impact of screening and other experimental tumor studies. Cancer Treat Rev 1975; 2:1-31.

[25]   Norton L, Simon R, Brereton HD, Bogden AE. Predicting the course of Gompertzian growth. Nature 1976; 264:542-5.

[26]   Simpson-Herren L, Sanford AH, Holmquist JP. Cell population kinetics of transplanted and metastatic Lewis lung carcinoma. Cell Tissue Kinet 1974; 7:349-6.

CHAPTER 10

Breast Cancer: 1. Hormonal Interventions: A New Era Begins

Pierre R. Band[*]

Department of Medicine, McGill University, Montreal, Canada

Abstract: In the 1950s and 1960s, the treatment of metastatic breast cancer in women consisted of hormonal ablative or additive procedures. However, no tests were available to predict patients' response; as a result, about 60% to 70% of the women who underwent these endocrine procedures failed to respond. The discovery of the estrogen receptor enabled clinicians to select those women with breast cancer most likely to respond to hormonal procedures. Response to endocrine therapy occurred in about 60% of women with estrogen receptor rich tumors, as opposed to 8% in women with estrogen receptor poor tumors. Of added importance, assay of the estrogen receptor in the primary breast tumor was found to be predictive of response to endocrine therapy in women who subsequently developed disease recurrence. Tamoxifen, an anti-estrogenic compound synthesized in Great Britain, inhibits the binding of estrogen to the estrogen receptor. Tamoxifen underwent extensive fundamental and clinical investigations and became the standard form of endocrine therapy for breast cancer for over a quarter of a century.

Keywords: Breast cancer, endocrine therapy, estrogen receptors, tamoxifen.

FROM THE MATTERHORN TO ESTROGEN RECEPTORS, OR LOOK FOR THE ALTERNATIVE

As discussed in Chapter 2, the treatment of metastatic breast cancer in the 1950s and 1960s consisted of hormonal ablative or additive procedures. In general, first-line treatment in premenopausal and perimenopausal women was bilateral ovariectomy or ovarian irradiation, whereas bilateral adrenalectomy, hypophysectomy or pharmacologic doses of estrogens were used in women five years or more past menopause. In women who were two to five years

---

*Address correspondence to Pierre R. Band: Faculty of Medicine, McGill University, Montreal, Quebec H3G 1Y6, Canada; E-mail: pierre.band@gmail.com

postmenopausal, androgens, bilateral adrenalectomy or hypophysectomy were considered [1-3]. Unfortunately, no tests were available to guide the clinician in recommending hormonal procedures to patients who were likely to respond. As a result only 30% to 40% of the patients undergoing such treatment responded, and the majority was subjected to operative complications or side effects of medication without therapeutic benefit. Patients with good results from primary hormonal treatment had about a 30% to 40% chance of responding to second line hormonal therapy; patients who did not have good results had negligible responses to further hormonal therapy.

Secondary endocrine therapy, which included surgical procedures or various hormones (androgens, progestins, corticosteroids) became restricted to responders to first-line hormonal treatment. Selecting the appropriate modality for a specific patient was an intricate "art of medicine" decision: "Thus, for each patient the most suitable methods of endocrine therapy are selected in a particular sequence depending mainly on the age of the patient, the urgency of the symptoms, the site of metastasis, the history of previous hormonal response, and the general condition of the patient [3]". This situation was to be changed by an organic chemist, Dr. Elwood Jensen, whose work on the mechanism of action of steroid hormones opened a new era in molecular and cancer endocrinology.

During his stay in Switzerland as a post-doctoral fellow in steroid biochemistry in the laboratory of Leopold Ruzicka (1887-1976), recipient of the Nobel Prize in Chemistry in 1939, Jensen climbed the Matterhorn and was surprised that a novice could succeed while expert mountaineers had repeatedly failed. The Matterhorn was the last major European peak to be conquered, an event that occurred in 1865; until then, most attempts were made from the Italian side, as the Swiss side was considered impossible to climb. A British engraver and passionate alpinist named Edward Whymper (1840-1911) had himself been unsuccessful in attempting the climb from the Italian side. He decided to try the Swiss side and finally reached the Matterhorn summit [4-6]. "The lesson of the alternative approach lived on to have an important influence in the discovery of the estrogen receptor [4]". Jensen left Switzerland to join the Charles Huggins Laboratory. He was fascinated when Huggins showed him "how minute amounts of estradiol administered to immature rats can cause spectacular growth of the uterus and other reproductive organs, and I resolved to find out just how it did it [4]". At that time, the prevalent thinking was that steroid hormones acted through enzymatic processes. For Jensen, however, "it seemed that one might obtain valuable clues by taking an alternative approach. Rather than asking what the hormone does to the tissue, one could find out what the tissue does with the hormone [4]".

In 1959, researchers in England had first noted the selective uptake and retention of tritium-labeled hexoestrol, a synthetic estrogen, in estrogen-responsive tissue of female goats and sheep [7]. At the time, tritium-labeled compounds were not readily available and research laboratories needed to synthesize their own. Herbert Jacobson, the co-discoverer of the estrogen receptor [5], developed a method to determine tritium in blood and tissues [8]. Tritium-labeled estradiol of very high specific activity was synthesized [5, 9], which, on administration to female rats was found to selectively accumulate in estrogen target tissues, suggesting the presence of a specific binding substance in those tissues [9, 10]. It was also noted that tritiated estradiol in uterine tissue was not chemically changed [11]. Thus "the tissues sensitive to stimulation by estrogens seemed to contain a specific component that binds estradiol without changing it chemically [4]". Jensen subsequently observed that the effect of estrogen on uterine growth was inhibited by an antiestrogen compound, providing the first evidence that binding of estradiol to the receptor was linked to its biological action [12]. Based on this and other experimental evidence, Jensen and co-workers proposed that the interaction of the hormone with its target tissue involved a two-step mechanism. Estradiol first binds to a cytosolic "uptake receptor" that becomes converted into a "biochemical functional form"; this "activated" estrogen-receptor complex translocates into the cell nucleus, binds to chromatin and triggers a chain of biochemical reactions leading in particular to cell proliferation [9, 13, 14]. This two-step process was subsequently shown to be a common mechanism of steroid hormone action [5, 9]. Another major contribution of Jensen's laboratory was the development of a monoclonal antibody to the estrogen receptor that eventually resulted in an immunoassay for estrogen receptor in breast cancer tissue [5, 9].

ESTROGEN RECEPTOR AND BREAST CANCER

In 1961, clinical investigators in England administered tritium-labeled hexoestrol to breast cancer patients prior to performing a bilateral adrenalectomy and ovariectomy. Women who responded to the treatment accumulated higher levels of the synthetic estrogen in their metastases than those who failed to respond [15]. It was also shown in rats bearing the 7, 12-dimethylbenzanthracene (DMBA)-induced hormone-dependent mammary tumor that tritium-labeled estradiol accumulated in the nuclei of tumor cells as well as in the tumor of animals responding to ovariectomy [16, 17].

Jensen and colleagues subsequently reported that the affinity of tritium-labeled estradiol for uterine receptor sites *in vitro* was similar to that observed *in vivo*, and demonstrated the presence of estrogen receptors in the nuclei of DMBA-induced mammary tumor cells [18]. They proposed: "One application, which suggests itself, for demonstrating whether or not a tissue contains estrogen receptors is the prediction of the response of human breast cancer to adrenalectomy [18]". Consequently, a clinicial trial was initiated to correlate the presence of estrogen receptors in tumors of women having breast cancer with responses to adrenalectomy. The preliminary results of the trial, reported in 1971 in 33 patients with advanced breast cancer, suggested that "patients whose breast cancers lack the estrogen-receptor substance have very little chance of responding to endocrine therapy. Of those patients who possess estrogen-binding proteins, some, but not all, will benefit from such treatment [19]". Of particular importance, the study also included 51 patients from whom tumor tissue was taken from the mastectomy specimen to characterize the primary tumor in terms of estrogen-receptor content "for future correlation with the response to endocrine therapy in those patients in which the cancer might recur [19]". In follow-up reports, the levels of estrogen receptors were correlated with the response to endocrine therapy in patients with advanced breast cancer. Tumor specimens were classified into estrogen-receptor rich and estrogen-receptor poor. Response to endocrine therapy was noted in 63% of the former category and only 3% of the latter. Furthermore, primary breast tumor specimens were analysed in 15 patients who later developed disease recurrence; three out of four women with estrogen-receptor rich tumor responded to endocrine therapy compared to one of 11 with estrogen-receptor poor tumors [20, 21].

In 1974, an international workshop was held under the auspices of the National Cancer Institute Breast Cancer Task Force, at which results of 14 different laboratories were reviewed using common clinical evaluation criteria. In patients with estrogen-receptor positive tumors, response to endocrine therapy ranged between 55% and 60%, compared to 8% in patients with estrogen-receptor negative tumors [22]. A subsequent consensus-development meeting on steroid receptors in breast cancer held in 1979 confirmed and strengthened the conclusions of the 1974 workshop; in addition, a recommendation was made that the primary tumor be assayed for estrogen receptor "so that the assay information will be available when needed at the time of disseminated disease [23]".

Twenty years before, in 1958, when Jensen first reported his studies with tritium-labeled estrogens in rats at the International Congress of Biochemistry in Vienna, only 5 persons had attended, 3 of them other speakers. His session "conflicted with a plenary session where 1,000 people were (there) to hear how estradiol . . . doesn't work. So that's the background of estrogen receptor [6]".

TAMOXIFEN

Tamoxifen (ICI 46,474) is a synthetic triphenylethylene derivative developed by researchers at Imperial Chemical Industries Ltd. in the United Kingdom. The compound, which was found to have antiestrogenic properties and to prevent implantation of the fertilized ova in female rats [24, 25], was considered as a potential contraceptive. In view of its antiestrogenic effects, preliminary clinical trials in patients with advanced breast cancer were undertaken in the United Kingdom with promising results [26-28].

Imperial Chemical Industries Ltd. bought Stuart Pharmaceuticals to develop a marketing and sales effort in the United States. First located in Pasadena, California, Stuart Pharmaceuticals was moved to Wilmington, Delaware, in 1973. The company was mainly involved with cardiovascular compounds.

LOIS TRENCH

Lois Trench (Fig. **10.1**) was a biochemist at the National Cancer Institute when she saw a newspaper advertisement placed by ICI Imperial Chemical Industries-Americas, Inc. During her job interview in 1973, the Director of the Research Department kicked a stack of paper into the corner of the room and said: "One day this will have to be sent down to the National Cancer Institute for testing". When

Trench was hired she reminded the Research Director: "You had talked about a drug to send to the National Cancer Institute. I worked there and I am familiar with their system. Do you mind if I take a look at it?" She looked through the documents, found that it was a very interesting compound and went back to the Director asking his permission to make a few phone calls. One of those calls was to Dr. Paul P. Carbone (1931-2002) then Chief of the Medicine Branch at the National Cancer Institute [29].

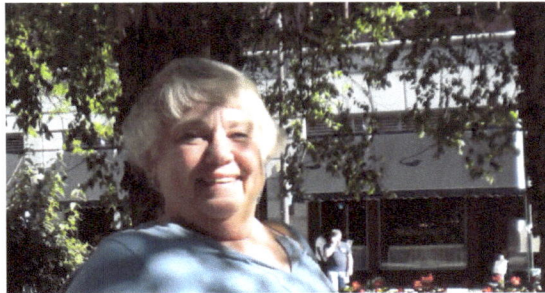

Figure 10.1: Lois Trench. Photo taken by the author; Philadelphia, 2011. Author's collection.

Around that time, she received calls from a young investigator by the name of Craig Jordan, then a fellow at the Worcester Foundation for Biomedical Research in Shrewsbury, Massachusetts. He needed tamoxifen citrate, which she sent. He also needed $2,000 to purchase rats for his experiments. Trench went to her Director, who refused to allocate the funds as tamoxifen was not on the schedule and there was no budget for it. The president of the Company also refused to grant any financial support. Trench asked permission to talk to the president: "I was 25 at the time, and when our discussion ended the President told me: 'What you want is seed money' and he gave me 10,000 dollars. That was the start of the development of tamoxifen in North America [29]".

Lois Trench became the drug monitor for tamoxifen and beyond doubt the catalyst for the fundamental and clinical investigation of this compound in North America.

THE AUTHOR GETS INVOLVED

When I returned to Canada from the United States, Carbone, who in addition to his work at the National Cancer Institute had become the ECOG chairman, asked me to chair the ECOG breast cancer committee. I met Trench in a small hotel board room where she had convened the breast cancer committee chairmen of a few cooperative oncology groups to seek their collaboration in developing clinical trials of tamoxifen. I told her of my interest and wrote a Phase II protocol for advanced breast cancer. It was planned as an international study involving Canada, the United States and Europe. The clinicians participating in the study were Lucien Israël in Paris, Harvey Lerner in Philadelphia and Pierre Band in Edmonton. Although the study was not registered with the ECOG, all three investigators were ECOG members (Fig. **10.2**: names in bold and underlined).

As it happened, I treated the first breast cancer patient with tamoxifen in North America. We were also the first in North America to show a correlation between tamoxifen response and estrogen-receptor positivity; the response rate was 69% in patients with estrogen-positive tumors, but no responses were observed in estrogen-receptor negative cases. The last sentence of the publication read: "The high degree of correlation observed between response rate and positive ER (estrogen receptor) assay suggests the value of this test as a means to select patients for tamoxifen treatment [30]". This international study became a major part of the new drug application submission that led to the U.S. Food and Drug Administration's approval for the use of tamoxifen in advanced breast cancer, granted in December 1977.

Lerner's clinic in Philadelphia was rather unusual; it had a live owl in the bathroom! The majority of his patients were poor, many living on welfare. Before tamoxifen was marketed, officials from Stuart Pharmaceuticals in Wilmington asked his opinion on how much a tamoxifen pill should cost. His reply was that they should see his patients, which they did. At the end of a long after-hours visit to Lerner's clinic and interviews with his patients, the Stuart Pharmaceuticals representatives told Lerner: "We will have to reduce the price drastically", which they also did.

The Tamoxifen Trio (Trench, Lerner and Band), as the author called it, reminisced about these events one memorable evening in November 2011 in Philadelphia, where the story began almost 40 years before.

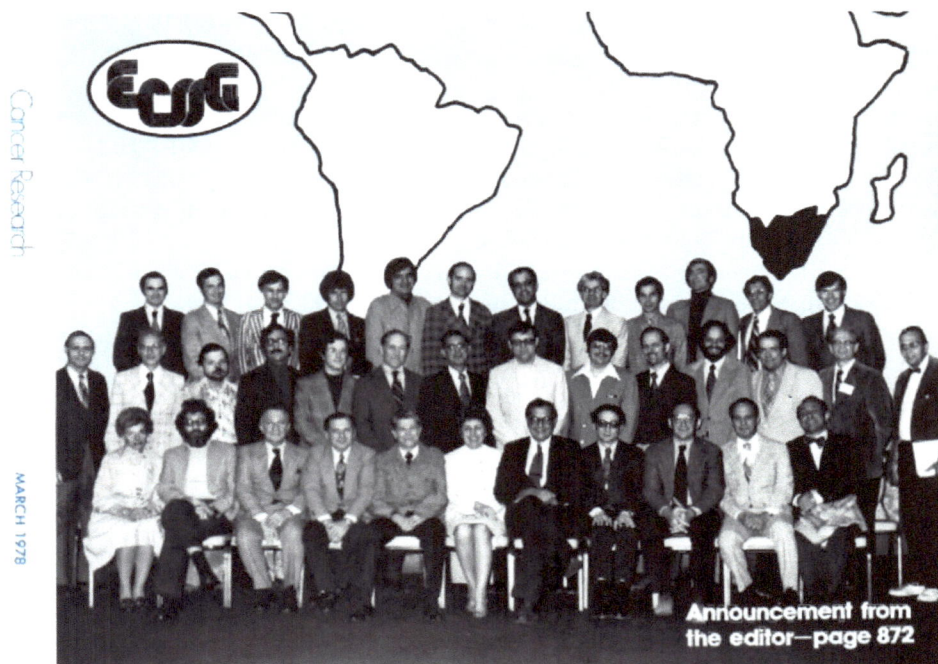

Figure 10.2: Photo kindly provided to the author by the Publications Department of the American Association for Cancer Research, Inc. From left to right: first row: Wolter J., Regelson W., Greenspan E., Colsky J, Shnider B., Grifone P., Carbone P., Zelen M., Cohen M., Brodsky I., **Israël L.**; second row: Sartiano G., Falkson G, Levitt M., Oken M., Straus M., Lenhard P., Tobin M., Marsh J., DeConti R., Costello W., Zucker S., Silberg R., Mittelman A., Lewis J.; third row: Stolbach.L, Creech R., Brodovsky H., Cunningham T., Kaplan B., DeWys W., Mansour E., Oberfield R., Bennett J., **Lerner H.**, **Band P.**, Klaassen D.

Tamoxifen became the standard form of endocrine therapy for breast cancer for over a quarter of a century. Tamoxifen was also found to produce results equivalent to ovarian ablation in premenopausal women with breast cancer [31]. Aminogluthetimide, a first generation aromatase inhibitor that is no longer used, had previously been shown to give results similar to surgical adrenalectomy in patients with metastatic breast cancer [32-34]. These effects of tamoxifen and of aminogluthetimide mark the beginning of what the author calls the "medicalization" of solid tumor therapy.

REFERENCES

[1]   Nathanson IT, Kelley RM. Hormonal treatment of cancer. N Engl J Med 1952; 246:135-45.
[2]   Kennedy BJ. Endocrine therapy of breast cancer. JAMA 1967; 200:971-2.

[3] Stoll BA. Hormonal management of advanced breast cancer. Br Med J 1969; 2:293-7.

[4] Jensen EV. From chemical warfare to breast cancer management. Nature Med 2004; 10:1018-21.

[5] Jensen EV, Jacobson HI, Walf AA, Frye CA. Estrogen action: a historic perspective on the implications of considering alternative approaches. Physiol Behav 2010; 99:151-62.

[6] Moore DD. A conversation with Elwood Jensen. Annu Rev Physiol 2012; 74:1–11.

[7] Glascock RF, Hoekstra WG. Selective accumulation of tritium-labelled hexoestrol by the reproductive organs of immature female goats and sheep. Biochem J; 1959; 72:673-82.

[8] Jacobson HI, Gupta GN, Fernandez C, Hennix S, Jensen EV. Determination of tritium in biological material. Arch Biochem Biophys 1960; 86:89-93.

[9] DeSombre ER. Estrogens, receptors and cancer: the scientific contributions of Elwood Jensen. Prog Clin Biol Res. 1990; 322:17-29.

[10] Jensen EV, Jacobson HI. Fate of steroid estrogens in target tissues. In "Biological Activities of Steroids in Relation to Cancer". Pincus G, Vollmer EP (eds), New York: Academic Press, 1960 pp 161-74.

[11] Jensen EV, Jacobson HI. Basic guides to the mechanism of estrogen action. Recent Prog Hormone Res 1962; 18:387-414.

[12] Jensen EV. Mechanism of estrogen action in relation to carcinogenesis. Proc Can Cancer Conf 1965; 6:143-65.

[13] Jensen EV, Suzuki T, Kawashima T, Stumpf WE, Jungblut PW, DeSombre ER. A two-step mechanism for the interaction of estradiol with rat uterus. Proc Natl Acad Sci USA 1968; 59:632-8.

[14] Jensen EV, DeSombre ER. Estrogen-receptor interaction. Science 1973; 182:126-34.

[15] Folca PJ, Glascock RF, Irvine WT. Studies with tritium-labelled hexœstrol in advanced breast cancer. Comparison of tissue accumulation of hexoestrol with response to bilateral adrenalectomy and oophorectomy. Lancet 1961; 2:796-8.

[16] King RJB, Cowan DM, Inman DR. The uptake of [6, 7-^{3}H] oestradiol by dimethylbenzanthracene-induced rat mammary tumours. J Endocrin 1965; 32:83-90.

[17] Mobbs BG. The uptake of tritiated oestradiol by dimethylbenzanthracene-induced mammary tumours of the rat. J Endocrinol 1966; 36:409-14.

[18] Jensen EV, DeSombre ER, Jungblut PW. Estrogen receptors in hormone-responsive tissues and tumors. In "Endogenous Factors Influencing Host-Tumor Balance". Wissler RW, Dao TL, Wood S Jr (Eds), Chicago: University of Chicago Press, 1967; pp 15-30.

[19] Jensen EV, Block GE, Smith S, Kyser K, DeSombre ER. Estrogen receptors and breast cancer response to adrenalectomy. Natl Cancer Inst Monogr 1971; 34:55-70.

[20] Jensen EV. Estrogen receptors in hormone-dependent breast cancers. Cancer Res 1975; 35 (11 Part 2):3362-4.

[21] Jensen EV, Smith S, DeSombre ER. Hormone dependency in breast cancer. J Steroid Biochem 1976; 7:911-7.

[22] McGuire WL. Current status of estrogen receptors in human breast cancer. Cancer 1975: 36 (Suppl 2):638-44.

[23] DeSombre ER, Carbone PP, Jensen EV, *et al*. Special report. Steroid receptors in breast cancer. N Engl J Med 1979; 301:1011-2.

[24] Harper MJK, Walpole AL. Contrasting endocrine activities of *cis* and *trans* isomers in a series of substituted triphenylethylenes. Nature 1966; 212:87.

[25]   Harper MJK, Walpole AL. A new derivative of triphenylethylene: effect on implantation and mode of action in rats. J Reprod Fertil 1967; 13:101-19.

[26]   Cole MP, Jones CTA, Todd IDH. A new anti-oestrogenic agent in late breast cancer. An early clinical appraisal of ICI 46,474. Br J Cancer 1971; 25:270-5.

[27]   Ward HWC. Anti-oestrogen therapy for breast cancer: a trial of tamoxifen at two dose levels. Br Med J 1973; 1:13-14.

[28]   O'Halloran MJ, Maddock PG. I.C.I 46,474 in breast cancer. J Irish Med Assoc 1974; 67:38-39.

[29]   Author's interview with Lois Trench.

[30]   Lerner HJ, Band PR, Israel L, Leung BS. Phase II study of tamoxifen: report of 74 patients with stage IV breast cancer. Cancer Treat Rep 1976; 60:1431-5.

[31]   Buchanan RB, Blamey RW, Durrant KR, *et al*. A randomized comparison of tamoxifen with surgical oophorectomy in premenopausal patients with advanced breast cancer. J Clin Oncol 1986; 4:1326-30.

[32]   Griffiths CT, Hall TC, Saba Z, Barlow JJ, Nevinny HB. Preliminary trial of aminoglutethimide in breast cancer. Cancer 1973; 32:31-7.

[33]   Santen RJ, Lipton A, Kendall J. Successful medical adrenalectomy with aminoglutethimide. Role of altered drug metabolism. JAMA 1974; 230:1661-5.

[34]   Santen RJ. Suppression of estrogens with aminogluthetimide and hydrocortisone (medical adrenalectomy) as treatment of advanced breast carcinoma: a review. Breast Cancer Res Treat 1981; 1:183-202.

"Clearly, the time has come to move nonhormonal chemotherapy into the forefront of the therapy of metastatic breast cancer." Dr. Steven K. Carter.

"It's not that Canadians are conservatives, they just don't want to be the first to do things." Heard by the author many years ago in a radio interview of Laurence J. Peter, co-author of The Peter Principle: Why Things Always Go Wrong.

CHAPTER 11

Breast Cancer: 2. A Paradigm for Solid Tumor Chemotherapy

Pierre R. Band[*]

Department of Medicine, McGill University, Montreal, Canada

Abstract: In the early 1960s, breast cancer was considered to be poorly responsive to chemotherapy. However, several agents, in particular methotrexate, vincristine, 5-fluorouracil, cyclophosphamide, an alkylating agent synthesized in Germany, and prednisone were found to be active in women with metastatic breast cancer. These five drugs were then used in advanced breast cancer in a combination referred to as the "Cooper regimen" that triggered a number of studies using quadruple and quintuple chemotherapeutic drug combinations which induced response rates superior to therapy with single agents. These results led to the integration of combination chemotherapy into a combined modality approach, epitomized by modern 'adjuvant' chemotherapy. A first randomized study comparing long-term postoperative single drug chemotherapy to a placebo led to improved survival in a subset of patients. Superior results were subsequently achieved with postoperative combination chemotherapy. The historical development of these approaches is described.

Keywords: Breast cancer, single agent chemotherapy, combination chemotherapy, postoperative ('adjuvant') chemotherapy.

INTRODUCTION

In the early 1960s, one of the great pioneers of medical oncology, David Karnofsky, listed breast cancer under the malignancies that are poorly responsive to chemotherapy [1]. Within a decade, breast cancer would become a paradigm for solid tumor chemotherapy. What accounted for that accomplishment within such a short time?

*Address correspondence to Pierre R. Band: Faculty of Medicine, McGill University, Montreal, Quebec H3G 1Y6, Canada; E-mail: pierre.band@gmail.com

SINGLE AGENT CHEMOTHERAPY

We have previously encountered two drugs that have changed the outlook of childhood acute leukemia: methotrexate and vincristine. The drugs were later shown to induce objective responses in over 20% of patients with metastatic breast cancer [2, 3]. Now let's meet two other compounds, among the oldest and, as it turned out, among the most useful chemotherapeutic agents: 5-fluorouracil and cyclophosphamide.

5-fluorouracil

5-fluorouracil (5-FU) was synthesized by Dr. Charles Heidelberger (1920-1983) at the McArdle Memorial Laboratory in Madison, Wisconsin [4]. It was designed "on a purely rational basis, its mode of action predicted in advance, and following synthesis and testing, was developed into a clinically useful drug that exerts its action as predicted [5]." The idea of creating an antitumor agent similar to uracil came from a study reporting a higher uptake of labeled uracil into a rat hepatoma than into normal liver cells. Thymidine, an essential building block of DNA, differs from uracil in having a methyl group instead of a hydrogen atom on the 5-carbon atom. The reasoning was that replacing the hydrogen atom of uracil on carbon-5 with a fluorine atom would lead to a potent analogue that might interfere with the synthesis of DNA. It was also known that substitution with a fluorine atom produces profound modifications of biological effects; for instance "such a substitution converts acetic acid to fluoroacetic acid and thus changes salad dressing into a commercial rat poison [6]!" The drug was active against a spectrum of experimental animal tumors, including the L1210 model [7], and a preliminary clinical study was initiated [8]. Results of subsequent clinical trials indicated that 5-fluorouracil induced beneficial responses against a number of tumor types, particularly colon cancer, other gastrointestinal malignancies, and breast cancer [3, 9-11]. Despite these successes, Heidelberger's satisfaction was mixed with frustration: "Whatever gratification I may feel from this limited success is far exceeded by the frustration caused by the fact that 5-FU does *not* favorably affect the majority of patients in whom it is tried. This frustration, compounded by the fact that several of my good friends have died after failing on this drug, serves as a continuing spur to try to do much better [6]."

Like several of his good friends, Charles Heidelberger died "as the victim of the disease to which he devoted essentially all of his professional life [12]."

Cyclophosphamide

The alkylating agent cyclophosphamide was synthesized in Germany [13]. The bis-β-chloroethyl group of mechlorethamine was bound to a phosphamide ring, converting it to an inert substance requiring enzymatic and chemical transformation into the active compound within the body [14, 15]. "In the beginning was the idea; Druckrey was the first in proposing to use a highly reactive drug as a 'prodrug' or '*latent drug*' in a chemically *masked*, inactive 'transport form'; this should be converted by specific enzymes into the active form in the tumor cell [15]." The pharmacological, experimental and clinical studies of cyclophosphamide, first undertaken in Germany, were soon initiated in other countries [16-20].

Cyclophosphamide is active against a broad spectrum of experimental animal tumors [21, 22]: "Among 1,000 selected compounds and antibiotics tested against all or portions of the tumor spectrum (33 tumors), cytoxan was the most effective, having a marked inhibitory to complete inhibitory effect on 26 out of 33 tumors [23]." Similarly, cyclophosphamide is effective against a wide range of hematologic and solid tumors in humans, including breast cancer [20, 24-28].

Clinical trials in childhood acute leukemia and lymphomas have pointed the way to the increased effectiveness of combination over single agent chemotherapy. With the availability of four non-hormonal agents each individually active, the time had come to develop combination chemotherapy for breast cancer.

COMBINATION CHEMOTHERAPY

Combination chemotherapy was pioneered by Dr. Ezra Greenspan (1919-2004). Starting in 1960, he treated 40 women with advanced metastatic breast cancer with a combination of methotrexate and an alkylating agent, Thio-TEPA; 35 of the women had received prior hormone therapy [29]. An overall response rate (complete and partial) was seen in 15 cases (43 %). These impressive results, similar to those of hormonal treatment in less advanced cases, were not appreciated at their true value; Greenspan was ahead of his time. A different fate was met by a 1969 abstract reporting major activity of a combination of cyclophosphamide, methotrexate, 5-fluorouracil, vincristine and prednisone, acronym CMFVP, in hormone-resistant breast cancer [30]. This combination was initiated in 1965 by Dr. Richard Cooper, who had a large oncology practice at the Buffalo General Hospital in Buffalo, New York. "The best response to single agents was only about 20%. This meant to me that 80% of the patients were getting worse. So I thought that it would be worthwhile to try drugs that did not have much in the way of overlapping toxicity and I combined the five drugs. I gave full doses of vincristine and prednisone, and about 80% of the full dose of the other 3 drugs. The first results were dramatic with tolerable toxicity, and it took off from there. What I did sort of became standard [31]." This therapy, referred to as the "Cooper regimen", triggered a number of clinical trials of combination chemotherapy in breast cancer from a medical oncology community that had considerably evolved since Greenspan's pioneering study. "Quadruple and quintuple drug chemotherapy in breast cancer patients was an outgrowth of the 1969 report by Cooper [32]." The non-randomized and randomized trials of four and five drug combinations in women with metastatic breast cancer, reviewed in 1974 [32], resulted in an overall response rate of 50%. Clearly, these results were superior to those for single agent chemotherapy and for hormonal treatments in unselected breast cancer patients. These achievements led to a radical change in therapeutic approaches to solid tumors and to the integration of chemotherapy into combined modality regimens epitomized by the breakthrough of surgical "adjuvant" chemotherapy.

The recognition that "surgery and radiation therapy have reached a plateau in their ability to cure solid tumors [33]", and the realisation that combination chemotherapy produced at least a 50% response rate in some metastatic cancers, led the National Cancer Institute's Division of Cancer Treatment, set up in 1973, to propose the integration of chemotherapy into combined modality of solid tumors. "The Division of Cancer Treatment's proposed strategy for increasing cure rates in solid tumors involves integration of drugs into combined modalities for primary treatment [33]." In the conventional way of treating solid tumors, surgery and/or radiation therapy were used as primary treatments of loco-regional disease, whereas chemotherapy was considered for metastatic or advanced disease. Breast cancer therapy was representative of this approach. In that disease, hormonal manipulations were used for recurrent and metastatic disease, chemotherapy being reserved for late stages. In the new proposal, "new drugs and combinations would be tested in advanced disease and those showing positive results would move into primary treatment of disseminated disease. The optimal regimen evolved in this situation would then be integrated into a combined modality approach for primary treatment of local and regional disease [33]."

SURGICAL ADJUVANT CHEMOTHERAPY

Experimental and early clinical studies

The idea of using systemic agents in conjunction with surgery originated before its clinical application. Similarly, testing combination chemotherapy in metastatic disease for potential use in the adjuvant setting preceded the scheme for solid tumor therapy developed by the Division of Cancer Treatment.

In the 1950s, attention was drawn to the finding of malignant cells in the blood stream during surgery, raising the possibility of tumor dissemination caused by operative manipulation [34, 35]. Chemotherapy given after administration of a suspension of cancer cells into the portal vein of experimental animals reduced the percentage of "takes" in the liver [35]. Based on this evidence, chemotherapy was given for four consecutive days beginning on the day of operation, to 45 patients with malignant diseases [35]. The authors of this approach were acknowledged to "deserve credit for initiating and developing interest in the United States in the use of nitrogen mustard and Thio-TEPA at the time of surgical resection of gastrointestinal neoplasms [36]." However, it had been pointed out that an inverse relationship existed between the number of tumor cells and the effectiveness of chemotherapeutic agents [37, 38]. In a first experiment using the Mammary adenocarcinoma 755, tumor response to 6-mercaptopurine decreased with increasing tumor mass. Furthermore, partial surgical tumor excision plus 6-mercaptopurine induced complete tumor regression in 57% of the animals, whereas no response occurred with either form of treatment alone. It was concluded: "the potential value of administering postoperative chemotherapy as an adjunct to surgery . . . not only offers hope for cure of the microscopic metastases and inadvertent tumor 'seeding' in the so-called operable and potentially curable group of cancer patients, but also offers new hope for those cancer patients hitherto categorized as incurable [37]." That study was later extended to other experimental animal models and chemotherapeutic agents with the following comments: "It is apparent from the data presented that surgical excision and adjuvant chemotherapy represented a marked increase in tumor 'cure' rate over either therapeutic modality alone . . . Clinical trial with the combined therapeutic modalities would allow the 'early' cancer patient to receive conventional cancer therapy (operation) as well as chemotherapy under optimal conditions for effectiveness [38]." The reader will not have failed to note the words "combined therapeutic modalities."

We have previously discussed the formation of the first cooperative oncology groups by the Cancer Chemotherapy National Service Center and its Clinical Studies Panel. These organizations also planned for the use of chemotherapeutic agents in conjunction with surgery with the view of improving therapeutic results for cancer patients with early disease. An important aim at that time was also to "develop workable methods and techniques for therapeutic trials in cancer [36]." The initial studies, organized in 1956, were targeted against lung and stomach cancers [36]. The first adjuvant study in breast cancer began in 1957 and was reported by the Surgical Adjuvant Chemotherapy Breast Group, later known as the National Surgical Adjuvant Breast Project (NSABP) [39, 40]. The treatment schedule was mainly based on experimental animal data indicating that the growth of cancer cells injected into animals could be significantly decreased with chemotherapy [39]. Consequently, the chemotherapeutic agent was only given on 3 consecutive days, beginning on the day of surgery [39].

The rationale for this early adjuvant study did not take into consideration the experimental evidence pointing to the potential effect of chemotherapy on microscopic metastases [37, 38]. It is informative to quote reflections on the context that prevailed in the late 1950s when cooperative surgical adjuvant studies were first undertaken:

> There was a reluctance to accept prolonged cancer chemotherapy in
> the postoperative period since chemotherapy was viewed as non-

curative and toxic . . . Many were unwilling to subject their ☐well patients" to a prolonged, distressing and dubious prospect for cure. This attitude led to the utilization of a very abbreviated course of postoperative chemotherapy . . . Many believed, wrongly, that all cancer cells circulating in the blood would be killed by a very brief exposure to a cytotoxic agent; were dislodged from the primary tumor during operation and were the major reason for tumor recurrence and distant metastasis . . . The laboratory demonstration that, although a full course of cancer chemotherapy could not cure an animal with a large tumor burden, it could destroy established microfoci of malignant cells remaining after surgical removal of the primary tumor, was utilized to help obtain funding approval for this first adjuvant thiotepa clinical trial. However, the experimental laboratory findings were not integrated into the subsequent protocol design [41].

Recollections of the author

1. Melphalan

On returning to Canada from the United States, my first endeavor was to affiliate the University of Alberta in Edmonton, with the ECOG. We became the first Canadian organization joining this group. The second was to write a protocol for postoperative chemotherapy in women with Stage II breast cancer; the rational was based on the kinetics of tumor growth, discussed in Chapter 9, which pointed to the high probability of systemic micrometastases at the time of diagnosis. To eradicate these micrometastases, prolonged chemotherapy initiated soon after removal of the primary tumor would be needed. I intended to submit this project to the National Cancer Institute of Canada for a Clinical Research Associate Grant. At the time, the organization did not have a Clinical Trials Group. I was interviewed by a virologist and an immunologist who had no clue what I was talking about (the reverse was equally true!), and my application was rejected. Soon after, I received a phone call from Dr. William Regelson (1925-2002), who was a member of Holland's staff at Roswell Park Memorial Institute while I was there. Regelson had since moved to head the Division of Medical Oncology at the Medical College of Virginia, now Virginia Commonwealth University. He told me that Dr. Bernard Fisher, who had recently visited him, was keenly interested in surgical adjuvant studies of breast cancer and that I should get in touch with him. I sent the protocol to Fisher (Fig. **11.1**: letter; Fig. **11.2**: photo) and to Carbone (Fig. **11.3**: letter received; Fig. **11.2**: photo), who at the time was being approached to become the ECOG Chairman.

When Carbone became chairman of the ECOG he invited me to chair the Group's Breast Cancer Disease Oriented Committee and to pursue discussions with Fisher. I first met Fisher in his hotel room in Houston, Texas, on the occasion of the Congress of the International Union against Cancer in 1971. The room was fairly large, with all chairs and the bed covered with files and papers. Fisher was writing a paper. The hotel room had become the temporary office of a hard working-man who had to remove files from a chair so I could sit down. This was the beginning of the joint surgical adjuvant study between two of the earliest cooperative oncology groups, the ECOG and the NSABP. In my original protocol cyclophosphamide was compared to a placebo. Because cyclophosphamide causes hair loss, it was agreed to replace it with the drug melphalan (L-PAM). The protocol was ready to be finalized at an ECOG meeting held in Jasper Park, Alberta, in 1971 (Fig. **11.4**).

Dr. Bernard Fisher,
Professor and Director,
Laboratory of Surgical Research,
University of Pittsburgh,
School of Medicine,
Pittsburgh, Pennsylvania, 15213.

Dear Dr. Fisher:

     Enclosed is the proposed breast protocol with some modifications.

     A lot remains to be discussed, and I look forward to meeting you in Houston.

                        Yours sincerely,

PRB/am

Encl.

                        P. R. Band, M.D.,
                        Department of Medicine.

Figure 11.1: Letter to Dr. Bernard Fisher.

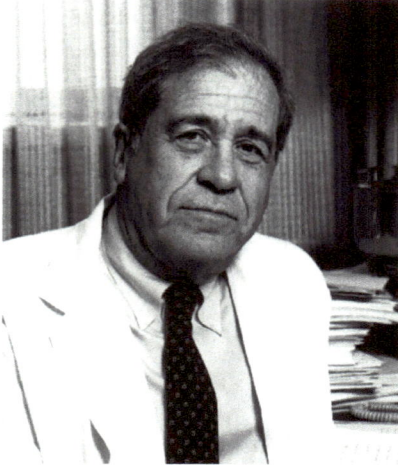

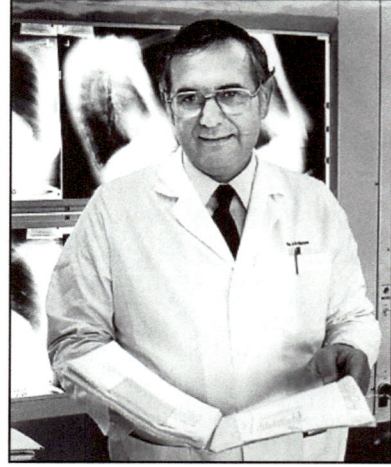

Figure 11.2: Left: Dr. Bernard Fisher. Source: http://www.225.pitt.edu/story/bernard-fisher-rethinking-cancer-care. Reproduced with Dr. Bernard Fisher's authorization. Right: Dr. Paul P. Carbone; courtesy of the Carbone Cancer Center, University of Madison, Wisconsin.

DEPARTMENT OF HEALTH, EDUCATION, AND WELFARE
PUBLIC HEALTH SERVICE
NATIONAL INSTITUTES OF HEALTH
BETHESDA, MARYLAND 20014

July 13, 1970

R.P. Band, M.D.
Department of Medicine
Clinical Sciences Building
The University of Alberta
Edmonton 61, Alberta

Dear Dr. Band:

I was most interested in reading your protocol and would be most anxious to participate in the discussion of an adjuvant breast cancer protocol.

As yet I have not heard from Dr. Shnider, but I will contact him directly.

Sincerely yours,

Paul P. Carbone, M.D.
Chief, Medicine Branch
National Cancer Institute

Figure 11.3: Letter from Dr. Paul Carbone.

A preliminary report on the results showed that in premenopausal women the difference in disease-free survival between the treated and control groups was highly significant [42].

1. Surgical Adjuvant Protocol with L-PAM (Phase II)
    (Dr. Band)
    A protocol was circulated to senior investigators for
    comments prior to the meeting. Before final activation
    of the protocol, provisions must be made for: (a) path-
    ology review (to be worked out with Dr. Friedell of the
    Breast Cancer Task Force); (b) formulation of drugs
    (approx. 2 months); (c) funding for Dr. Fisher; (d)
    new breast and pathology forms. Forms devised by Dr.
    B. Fisher will be looked at carefully and considered
    for immediate adoption. Post-operative radiation
    therapy has been excluded following unanimous decision
    by the Group. A final version of the protocol is being
    prepared by Drs. Fisher and Band. This study will be a
    combined effort of the ECOG and the National Surgery
    Adjuvant Breast Program.

Figure 11.4: Excerpt from the minutes of the ECOG meeting, Jasper Park, Alberta, June 1971.

In 1971, the same situation prevailed in Canada as in the United States in the 1950s: chemotherapy was met with suspicion, if not outright antagonism. I was treating breast cancer patients with adjuvant chemotherapy. To give toxic drugs to patients with metastatic cancer might perhaps be tolerated, but poisoning well women was, some thought, the act of a fool. I soon had most staff of the Cancer Center in Edmonton against me (there were exceptions), and the Director put pressure on the Dean of the Faculty of Medicine not to grant me tenure. Fortunately the Dean, a surgeon who had been operated on for colon cancer, paid no attention. These experiences are in no way unique; I have spoken to many colleagues of the pre-subspecialty era who faced similar opposition and rebuffs. Cancer medicine was no exception to the way innovations are received by many conservative thinkers in the medical establishment. This led me to write to the Executive Director of the National Cancer Institute of Canada in 1973: "The National Cancer Institute of Canada should shake its conservatism and support potential clinical investigators even if at times it turns out that the bet was made on the wrong horse. A more open attitude will have to prevail as the future will no doubt see the return to Canada of well-trained oncologists who will naturally rely on the help of the National Cancer Institute of Canada at the beginning of their career in this country."

2. CMF

The melphalan trial, the first randomized long-term surgical adjuvant chemotherapy study in breast cancer, used a single agent at a dose producing limited side effects. Fisher wanted to avoid the possibility of serious adverse reactions that might jeopardize future adjuvant studies. Since it was known that combination chemotherapy was likely to produce superior results, we initiated within the ECOG a study comparing a single agent to combination chemotherapy in women with metastatic breast cancer [43]. The combination, which used cyclophosphamide, methotrexate and 5-fluorouracil, was adapted from a phase II study carried out at the National Cancer Institute that induced responses in 17 of 25 patients (68%) with metastatic disease [44]. The single agent was melphalan, given at the same dose and schedule as in the adjuvant study. The purpose was to use the combination, if found to be superior, in the next generation of adjuvant trials (Fig. **11.5**). The result was highly significant, with a response rate of 53% for the combination that became known as CMF, compared to 20% for the single agent [43]. This study also illustrates the therapeutic approaches that were adopted by the Division of Cancer Treatment.

3. Combination Study (L-PAM)   (Drs. Canellos, Taylor and
    Band)
    Protocol for combination therapy of breast carcinoma
    previously untreated with chemotherapeutic agents (does
    not exclude previous hormonal additive or ablative therapy).
    This protocol will compare initially a three-drug com-
    bination (5FU-MTX-CYT) to L-PAM given at the dosage and
    schedule used in the Surgical Adjuvant Study.

    Fifty evaluable cases are required in each group--the
    less active regimen will be dropped in favor of a new
    combination. The aim of this study is to find a tol-
    erable and active drug combination for further evaluation
    in a large Phase III protocol in association with hormones,
    and in a future surgical adjuvant study, should the com-
    bination prove to be more active than L-PAM. The initial
    protocol will be prepared by Drs. Canellos and Taylor, and
    should be activated prior to the next ECOG meeting.

Figure 11.5: Excerpt from the minutes of the ECOG meeting, Jasper Park, Alberta, June 1971.

In 1972, Carbone informed Dr. Gianni Bonadonna (Fig. **11.6**) from the National Cancer Institute of Italy in Milan of the ECOG comparative trial of combination chemotherapy in breast cancer, as well as the joint NSABP-ECOG surgical adjuvant protocol. Bonadonna thought that the testing of CMF in the adjuvant setting would be important. Carbone agreed and a contract was drawn up with Bonadonna's Institution. Bonadonna then undertook a surgical adjuvant study comparing CMF to a placebo, with improved results compared to those of the NSABP-ECOG trial [45].

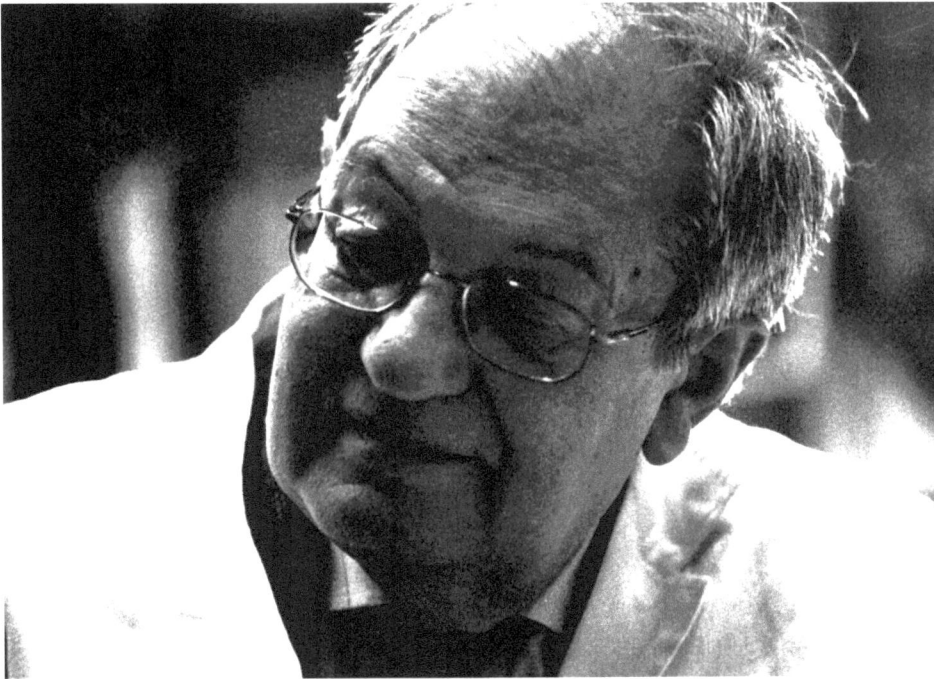

Figure 11.6: Dr. Gianni Bonadonna. Photograph kindly received from Dr. Bonadonna.

Both adjuvant studies had a precursor. In 1968, after noting the efficacy of CMFVP in women with advanced metastatic breast cancer, Cooper initiated a non-randomized study using the same combination post-mastectomy in patients at high risk of recurrence, those with four or more axillary lymph nodes involved with tumor. Regrettably, his study was published in 1979 [46], four years after the melphalan and CMF adjuvant studies [41, 44]. As a result, Cooper did not receive the recognition he deserved for having been the first to initiate a long-term adjuvant combination chemotherapy trial in breast cancer. "I was in practice and on my own, what I did was not part of a big national study and I did not have untreated controls. I gave the patients the best care they could get and it did not mean watching the natural history of the disease which I thought I already knew. Also, it made no sense to use a single drug when I knew that better results could be achieved with combination chemotherapy [31]."

The melphalan study was a model for the modern surgical "adjuvant" trials. The term "adjuvant", meaning ancillary or auxiliary, was properly applied to the initial trial aimed at eradicating circulating tumor cells dislodged during surgery. The term was no longer appropriate for studies with a curative intent aiming to destroy micrometastatic foci left after removal of the primary tumor. Unfortunately, the term remained entrenched in the cancer literature.

THE LAST NAIL IN THE COFFIN OF THE HUMORAL THEORY: AN INCURSION INTO SURGERY

In Chapter 2 we saw that after the lymphatic system was described, Descartes conceived the lymphatic theory of cancer; however, this theory was still akin to the humoral theory. Cancer was viewed as a local disease, spreading the lymphatic system before reaching the blood circulation. In the 1950s the standard surgical procedure for operable breast cancer was Dr. William Halsted's (1852-1922) radical mastectomy, generally followed by radiation therapy to the regional node-bearing areas. The concept on which this operation and the radiation therapy aspects are based had its roots in the lymphatic theory of cancer that originated in the 17th century. This notion persisted, owing to Virchow's view that regional lymph nodes acted as a barrier to tumor spread and Halsted's belief that cancer disseminated by continuity *via* the lymphatic system [47]. Three centuries passed before these concepts were challenged by Doctors Bernard Fisher and his brother Edwin, in an elegant series of experiments on the role of lymph nodes [48]. The Fishers concluded that lymph nodes were not a barrier to the spread of tumor cells, but indicators of the host-tumor relationships involved in cancer dissemination.

Their research not only cast new light on tumor biology, but also provided support to the notion derived from the study of tumor growth rates that breast cancer is largely a systemic disease at the time it is diagnosed, and consequently variations in local and regional therapy would be unlikely to affect survival [48]. Beginning in 1961, this hypothesis was tested in a series of carefully planned and methodical clinical trials by the NSABP, under Bernard Fisher's chairmanship of many years. The first study compared radical mastectomy with regional radiation therapy, the standard treatment at that time, to radical mastectomy alone [49]. A second study initiated in 1971 compared radical mastectomy alone to total (simple) mastectomy, with or without radiation therapy [50]. Subsequently, total mastectomy alone was compared to tumorectomy with or without radiation therapy [51]. None of these trials showed differences in overall survival, confirming that the hypothesis on which these studies were based was well founded.

As a result, women with breast cancer are now spared the disfiguring and psychological effects of radical mastectomy. Bernard Fisher will forever stand as one of the giants of oncology for his breakthrough work in breast cancer, ranging from biology to innovative therapy.

REFERENCES

[1]   KarnofskyDA. Chemotherapy of cancer and its present position in the management of neoplastic disease. In "Proceedings of the international symposium on chemotherapy of cancer." Plattner PA (Ed), New York, Elsevier, 1964, pp 3-17.

[2]   Mittelman A, Grinberg R, Dao T. Clinical experience with vincristine (NSC-67574) in advanced cancer of the breast. Cancer Chemother Rep 1964; 34:25-30.

[3]   Comparison of antimetabolites in the treatment of breast and colon cancer. Eastern Cooperative Group in Solid Tumor Chemotherapy. JAMA 1967; 200:770-8.

[4]   Heidelberger C, Chaudhuri NK, Danneberg P, *et al.* Fluorinated pyrimidines, a new class of tumour-inhibitory compounds. Nature 1957; 179: 663-6.

[5]   Heidelberger C. On the rational development of a new drug: the example of the fluorinated pyrimidines. Cancer Treat Rep 1981; 65 (Suppl 3):3-9.

[6]   Heidelberger C. Chemical carcinogenesis, chemotherapy: cancer's continuing core challenges -- G.H.A. Clowes Memorial Lecture. Cancer Res 1970; 30:1549-69.

[7]   Heidelberger C, Griesbach L, Montag BJ, *et al.* Studies on fluorinated pyrimidines. II. Effects on transplanted tumors. Cancer Res 1958; 18:305-17.

[8]   Curreri AR, Ansfield FJ, McIver FA, Waisman HA, Heidelberger C. Clinical studies with 5-Fluorouracil. Cancer Res 1958; 18:478-84.

[9]   Moertel CG, Reitemeier RJ, Hahn RG. Fluorinated pyrimidine therapy of advanced gastrointestinal cancer. Gastroenterology 1964; 46:371-8.

[10]   Heidelberger C, Ansfield FJ. Experimental and clinical use of fluorinated pyrimidines in cancer chemotherapy. Cancer Res 1963; 23:1226-43.

[11]   Ansfield FJ, Ramirez G, Mackman S, Bryan GT, Curreri AR. A ten-year study of 5-fluorouracil in disseminated breast cancer with clinical results and survival times. Cancer Res 1969; 29:1062-6.

[12]   Miller EC, Miller JA. Charles Heidelberger 1920-1983. Cancer Res 1983; 43:2382.

[13]   Arnold H, Bourseaux F. Synthese und abbau zytostatish wirksamer zyclischer N-Phosphamidester des bis (β-chloroäthyl-) amins. Angew Chem 1958; 70:539-44.

[14]   Arnold H, Bourseaux F, Brock N. Chemotherapeutic action of a cyclic nitrogen mustard phosphamide ester (B 518-ASTA) in experimental tumours of the rat. Nature 1958; 181:931.

[15]   Brock N. The history of the oxazaphosphorine cytostatics. Cancer 1996; 78:542-7.

[16]   Brock N. Zur pharmakologischen charakterisierung zyklischer N-lost-phosphamidester als krebs-chemotherapeutica. Arzneimittelforschung 1958; 8:1-9.

[17]   Arnold H, Bourseaux F, Brock NA. Neuartig krebs-chemotherapeutika aus der gruppe der zyklischen n-lost-phosphamidester. Naturwiss 1958; 45:64-6.

[18]   Brock N, Wilmanns H. Wirkung eines zyklischer N-lost-phosphamid esters auf experimentell erzeugte tumoren der ratte. Deut Med Wschr, 1958; 83:453-8.

[19]   Gross R, Lambers K. Erste erfahrungen in der behandlung maligner tumoren mit einen neuen n-lost-phosphamidester. Deut Med Wschr 1958; 83:458-62.

[20]   Coggins PR, Ravdin RG, Eisman SH. Clinical evaluation of a new alkylating agent : cytoxan (cyclophosphamide). Cancer 1960; 13:1254-60.

[21]   Clinical pharmacology and preliminary evaluation of cytoxan (cyclophosphamide). Cancer Treat Rep 1959; 3:9-11.

[22]   Lane M, Yancey ST. The effectiveness of cyclophosphamide (cytoxan) against well established transplanted rodent tumors. Cancer Res 1960; 20:1269-73.

[23]   Sugiura K, Schmid FA, Schmid MM. Antitumor activity of cytoxan. Cancer Res 1961; 21:1412-20.

[24]   Matthias JQ, Misiewicz JJ, Scott RB. Cyclophosphamide in Hodgkin's disease and related disorders. Br Med J 1960; 2:1837-40.

[25]   Fernbach DJ, Sutow WW, Thurman WG, Vietti TJ. Clinical evaluation of cyclophosphamide. A new agent for the treatment of children with acute leukemia. JAMA 1962; 182:30-7.

[26]   Burkitt D, Hutt MSR, Wright DH. The African lymphoma. Preliminary observations on response to therapy. Cancer 1965; 18:399-410.

[27]   Stoll BA, Matar JH. Cyclophosphamide in advanced breast cancer. Br Med J 1961; 2:283-6.

[28]   Carter SK, Livingston RB. Cyclophosphamide in solid tumors. Cancer Treat Rev 1975; 2:295-322.

[29]   Greenspan EM, Fieber M, Lesnick G, Edelman S. Response of advanced breast carcinoma to the combination of the antimetabolite, methotrexate, and the alkylating agent, thio-TEPA. J Mt Sinai Hosp NY 1963; 30:246-67.

[30]   Cooper RG. Combination chemotherapy in hormone resistant breast cancer. Proc Am Assoc Cancer Res 1969; 10:15.

[31]   Author's interview with Dr. Richard Cooper.

[32]   Broder LE, Tormey DC. Combination chemotherapy of carcinoma of the breast. Cancer Treat Rev 1974; 1:183-203.

[33]   Carter SK, Soper WT. Integration of chemotherapy into combined modality treatment of solid tumors. 1. The overall strategy. Cancer Treat Rev 1974; 1:1-13.

[34]   Engell HC. Cancer cells in the circulating blood; a clinical study on the occurrence of cancer cells in the peripheral blood and in venous blood draining the tumor area at operation. Acta Chir Scand Suppl 1955; 201:1-70.

[35]   McDonald GO, Livingston C, Boyles CF, Cole WH. The prophylactic treatment of malignant disease with nitrogen mustard and triethylenethiophosphoramide (ThioTEPA). Ann Surg 1957; 145:624-9.

[36]   Shimkin MB, Moore GE. Adjuvant use of chemotherapy in the surgical treatment of cancer. Plan of cooperative study. JAMA 1958; 167:1710-14.

[37]   Shapiro DM, Fugmann RA. A role for chemotherapy as an adjunct to surgery. Cancer Res 1957; 17:1098-1101.

[38]   Martin DS, Fugmann RA. Clinical implications of the interrelationship of tumor size and chemotherapeutic response. Ann Surg 1960; 151:97-100.

[39]   Breast adjuvant chemotherapy: effectiveness of thio-thepa (triethylenethiophosphoramide) as adjuvant to radical mastectomy for breast cancer. Surgical Adjuvant Chemotherapy Breast Group. Ann Surg 1961; 154:629-45.

[40]   Noer RJ. Adjuvant chemotherapy. Thio-Tepa with radical mastectomy in the treatment of breast cancer. Am J Surg 1963; 106:405-12.

[41]   Martin DS. The scientific basis for adjuvant chemotherapy. Cancer Treat Rev 1981; 8:169-89.

[42]   Fisher B, Carbone P, Economou SG, *et al.* L-Phenylalanine mustard (L-PAM) in the management of primary breast cancer. A report of early findings. N Engl J Med 1975; 292:117-22.

[43]   Canellos GP, Pocock SJ, Taylor SG III, Sears ME, Klaasen DJ, Band PR. Combination chemotherapy for metastatic breast carcinoma. Prospective comparison of multiple drug therapy with L-phenylalanine mustard. Cancer 1976; 38:1882-6.

[44]   Canellos GP, DeVita VT, Gold GL, Chabner BA, Schein PS, Young RC. Cyclical combination chemotherapy for advanced breast carcinoma. Br Med J 1974; 1:218-20.

[45]   Bonadonna G, Brusamolino E, Valagussa P, *et al.* Combination chemotherapy as an adjuvant treatment in operable breast cancer. N Engl J Med 1976; 294:405-10.

[46]   Cooper RG, Holland JF, Glidewell O. Adjuvant chemotherapy of breast cancer. Cancer 1979; 44:793-8.

[47]   Fisher B. The surgical dilemma in the primary therapy of invasive breast cancer: a critical appraisal. Curr Probl Srug. 1970; Oct:1-53.

[48]   Fisher B. Biological research in the evolution of cancer surgery: a personal perspective. Cancer Res 2008; 68:10007-20.

[49]   Fisher B, Slack NH, Cavanaugh PJ, Gardner B, Ravdin RG (and cooperating investigators). Postoperative radiotherapy in the treatment of breast cancer: results of the NSABP clinical trial. Ann Surg 1970; 172:711-32.

[50]   Fisher B. Cooperative clinical trials in primary breast cancer: a critical appraisal. Cancer 1973; 31:1271-86.

[51]   Fisher B, Bauer M, Margolese R, *et al.* Five-year results of a randomised clinical trial comparing total mastectomy and segmental mastectomy with or without radiation in the treatment of breast cancer. N Engl J Med 1985; 312:665-73.

"The cancer shell begins to crack". Dr. Pierre R. Band.

CHAPTER 12

Successes in Solid Tumor Chemotherapy: Three Key Examples

Pierre R. Band[*]

Department of Medicine, McGill University, Montreal, Canada

Abstract: The chemotherapy of solid tumors followed the path opened by breast cancer: the use of active single agents combined for greater effectiveness in advanced disease and for their potential role in combined modality regimens. By the end of the 1960s, over 20 chemotherapeutic drugs effective against various malignancies were available to investigate these approaches. The use of combination chemotherapy in epithelial ovarian cancer, small cell lung cancer and osteogenic sarcoma showed improved response rates and duration of remission compared to previously used single drugs. Postoperative combination chemotherapy improved the survival of patients with osteogenic sarcomas.

Keywords: Ovarian cancer, small cell lung cancer, osteogenic sarcoma.

INTRODUCTION

The chemotherapy of solid tumors, in general, followed the path opened by breast cancer: the search for active single agents that could be combined for more effectiveness in advanced disease and for their potential role when combined with other therapeutic modalities. By the end of the 1960s, over 20 chemotherapeutic drugs effective against various malignancies had become available to research clinicians for investigation [1]. The drugs included doxorubicin (adriamycin), developed at the Farmitalia Research Institute in Milan, Italy,which attracted particular interest because of its activity in a wide spectrum of malignancies. The drug is an antibiotic produced by a mutant of *Streptomyces peucetius*, an organism obtained from a soil sample taken near the Adriatic Sea, hence the name adriamycin [2, 3]. Initial Phase I and Phase II studies were carried out under the leadership of Dr. Gianni Bonadonna at the Italian National Cancer Institute in

*Address correspondence to Pierre R. Band:** Faculty of Medicine, McGill University, Montreal, Quebec H3G 1Y6, Canada; E-mail: pierre.band@gmail.com

Milan [4, 5]. In 1970, a large Phase II study was jointly undertaken by the Southwest Cancer Chemotherapy Study Group in the United States and Bonadonna's group in Italy in patients with disseminated cancer. In malignancies with at least 50 cases studied, responses of 30% or greater were observed in malignant lymphomas, sarcomas, bladder and testicular cancers, and 14% in lung cancer [6]. These findings were confirmed in a 1974 review of the literature that also reported responses in acute leukemias [7].

EPITHELIAL OVARIAN CANCER

Ovarian cancer consists mainly of epithelial tumors of various histopathologies. In the early 1970s, ovarian malignancy was the fourth leading cause of mortality from cancer in women [8]. The clinical onset of such tumors is insidious and by the time symptoms supervene over two-thirds of patients have disseminated intra-abdominal disease or extra-abdominal metastases [8]. Epithelial ovarian cancers are highly sensitive to chemotherapeutic agents. For many years, alkylating agents, including melphalan and cyclophosphamide, were the sole compounds with demonstrated activity; these agents were administered in advanced stages after surgery and radiation therapy, or when radiation therapy was deemed inadvisable, with response rates ranging from 40% to 60% and median survivals approaching two years [8, 9]. As new compounds were being tested, methotrexate, 5-fluorouracil, hexamethylmelamine, a drug derived from an alkylating agent but having a different mechanism of action, doxorubicin and cisplatin were shown to induce responses in epithelial ovarian cancers [10-16]. Greenspan was among the first to use combination chemotherapy in ovarian tumors [17], but the first study comparing combination chemotherapy to a single agent was undertaken ten years later. The results showed a significantly increased overall response rate for the combination, with twice as many complete remissions [18]. Doxorubicin and/or cisplatin based combinations led to further improvement in response rate and duration [19, 20].

The 1970s also witnessed the publication of surgical studies of critical consequences. A collective review showed that at least 13% and 23% of patients with clinical stage I and II ovarian cancers respectively had tumor involvement corresponding to stage III disease [21]. To minimize misclassification and allow for more accurate staging, surgery with careful abdominal and retroperitoneal exploration became the norm. As a consequence comparative evaluation of therapeutic interventions between different studies became more reliable.

Investigation of the relationship between the extent of surgical resection of intra-abdominal ovarian tumor and survival showed that survival was inversely related to the size of the residual tumor masses. For example, the mean survival time of patients with no residual tumor after surgery was 39 months, compared to 11 months for those with residual masses exceeding 1.5 cm. It was concluded that: "Surgical bulk resection is of little value unless all or nearly all gross tumor is excised [22]".

In fact, in a retrospective study of cytoreductive surgery in patients with massive intra-abdominal Burkitt's lymphoma who received postoperative chemotherapy, sustained complete remissions and long term survival were significantly associated with tumor removal of 90% or greater. Remission and survival rates were significantly lower and similar for patients with tumor resection of less than 90% and for those who did not undergo surgery. The authors concluded: "If the experience with Burkitt's lymphoma is relevant to other tumour systems then the most dramatic improvements in results with large tumours are likely to be gained by emphasizing initial cytoreduction, utilizing all therapeutic modalities to their maximum extent, rather than prolonged intensive chemotherapy programs which may have little chance of increasing the cure rate in tumours above a critical size [23]".

These studies, which herald a role for surgery as an adjuvant to chemotherapy, also remind us that lessons from the past should always be kept in mind. In the 1950s it was shown in experimental animal tumor systems that surgical reduction of tumor masses was associated with an improved chemotherapy cure rate: "The less the amount of tumor tissue, the greater the chemotherapeutic effect [24]".

SMALL CELL LUNG CANCER

Small cell lung cancer (SCLC) differs from the other common pathological types of lung malignancies. It is often widely disseminated by the time it is diagnosed, with frequent involvement of the bone marrow and the brain; the median survival of patients with extensive disease, receiving supportive care only, does not exceed four months [25, 26]. SCLC is also distinct in its marked sensitivity to radiation therapy and its responsiveness to a wide variety of chemotherapeutic agents. Although responses to loco-regional radiation therapy are not reflected in increased survival [26], radiation therapy plays an important role in the management of SCLC, particularly in the prophylaxis of brain metastases, as suggested by Dr. Heine Hansen (1938-2011) [27], which effectively reduces the frequency of this serious event [28].

In the past, radiation therapy or surgery were used as primary treatments of patients with limited clinical disease. The United Kingdom Medical Research Council conducted a randomized study comparing the outcomes of surgery and radiation therapy in patients deemed operable. With a follow-up of 10 years, survival rates after radical radiation therapy surpassed rates after complete surgical resection. Though superior, the dismal outcome after radical radiation therapy, a mean survival of ten months with only 26% of the treated patients alive at one year, 11% at two years, and 5% at five years, led the authors to conclude: "The extremely low proportion of surviving patients, even in the group receiving the more favourable treatment, indicates that neither of the treatment policies studied is really effective [29]". It is against this background that the effects of chemotherapy must be judged particularly in limited disease (confined to one hemithorax and draining lymph nodes, encompassed by a single radiotherapy port).

In the 1970s, there were eight to ten chemotherapeutic agents known to induce at least a 25% response rate in SCLC [30]; clinical trials with various combinations of these compounds were undertaken. In patients with extensive disease, a number of studies reported median survivals of six to nine months [31], a non-negligible improvement when compared to supportive care, reminiscent of the early results of chemotherapy in childhood acute leukemia.

In patients with limited disease, combination chemotherapy was generally given in association with radiation therapy to the primary tumor and brain [31, 32]. In a study of 108 patients, an overall median survival of one year was achieved [32], clearly superior to the results of radical radiation therapy alone [29]. In a report of long-term survival of patients treated in the 1970s with or without radiation therapy, the 10-year survival of 103 patients with limited disease was 10%. The authors concluded: "Patients with small-cell lung cancer beginning treatment with currently available combination chemotherapy with or without irradiation can be assured that the proposed therapy offers not only substantial prolongation of survival compared with supportive care alone but also a small chance of cure [33]". It should be added that these results also represented a twofold improvement compared to radical radiation therapy in cases deemed to be operable [29].

OSTEOGENIC SARCOMA

"Osteogenic sarcoma has not been effectively controlled either by primary amputation, radiotherapy, or a combination of the two . . . Within a year, 50% of the patients have died from their disease . . . Chemotherapy has had little practical value in osteogenic sarcoma . . . The prognosis of a patient with pulmonary metastases from osteogenic sarcoma is considered nearly hopeless, the mean survival being six months from the onset of pulmonary involvement [34]". This was the situation in 1972, when doxorubicin [34] and high dose methotrexate with leucovorin rescue [35] were shown to induce complete regressions in patients with osteogenic sarcoma and lung metastases. Dr. Norman Jaffe (Fig. **12.1**), a pediatrician who had joined the Sidney Farber Cancer Institute in 1966 from South Africa, his country of birth, gave the following account of these events:

> We were at a loss; we had no way to prevent the development of lung metastasis following an amputation. Farber, a very impressive, charismatic and very clever individual had invited Dr. Isaac Djerassi to one of the tumor board's meetings. Djerassi told us how high dose methotrexate with leucovorin rescue was active in children with non-Hodgkin's lymphomas and adults with lung cancer who appeared resistant to methotrexate. I was quite impressed and asked Farber's permission to follow the same approach in osteogenic sarcoma. I can remember his words: "Proceed, young man". And I proceeded! We had no institutional review boards at that time, no surveillance committee, nothing. All that was needed was the permission of the Chief [36].

The current scientific bureaucracy would do well to ponder on the effectiveness of this *modus operandi* for the swift performance of promising clinical trials.

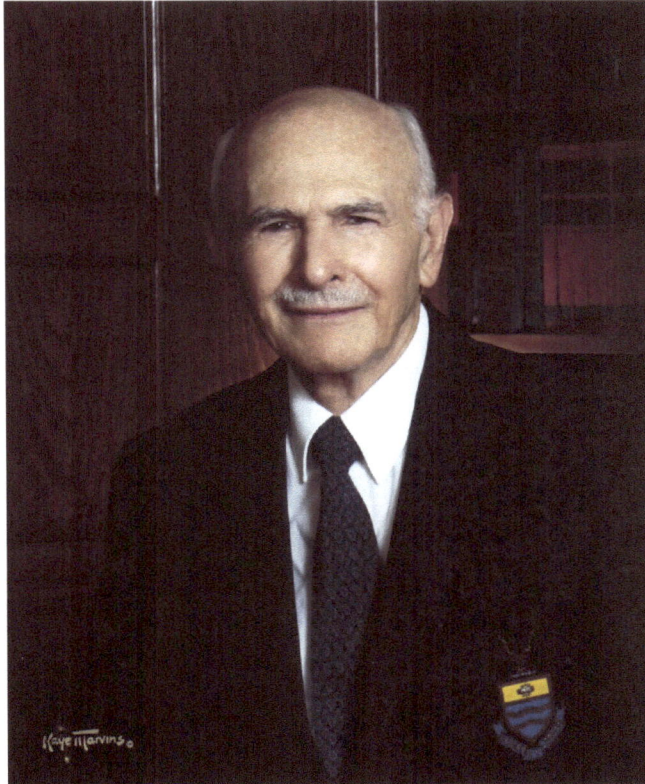

Figure 12.1: Dr. Norman Jaffe. Photograph kindly provided to the author by Dr. Jaffe.

"The first patient I treated with high dose methotrexate was a woman who had undergone a hemipelvectomy and who developed lung metastases within a few months. The response was dramatic; the lung metastases disappeared. She later gave birth to two healthy babies and to-day remains free of disease [36]". Jaffe later published a preliminary report on an adjuvant clinical trial of high-dose methotrexate and showed that 80% of "classic" osteogenic sarcoma historical controls, in whom local tumor control was achieved, developed pulmonary metastases within 18 months, whereas only one of the 12 (8%) receiving adjuvant therapy did the same [37]. Similar results on postoperative chemotherapy were published the same year by Cortes *et al*. with doxorubicin [38], and subsequently with a four-drug combination that included doxorubicin [39], suggesting "the exciting possibility that adjuvant chemotherapy has improved the prognosis in patients with osteogenic sarcoma [39]". All three studies used historical controls, one from the published literature, the other two from the same institutions where the adjuvant studies were performed. None of the historical control groups had shown changes in survival rates over the previous two decades.

THE HISTORICAL CONTROLS CONTROVERSY

Historical controls were selected on the basis of the following arguments: 1) The relative rarity of osteogenic sarcomas; 2) The dismal survival with amputation which remained relatively stable since the 1960s; 3) The promising results of chemotherapy in metastatic disease. The early results of the adjuvant studies, which showed significantly improved disease-free survival, were met with controversy. It was argued that differences in pre-treatment investigation to rule out lung metastases, imbalance between prognostic factors such as tumor size and grade between treated and control groups offered "no guarantee that the adjuvant chemotherapy groups were not more carefully selected with smaller tumors and a more extensive work-up to exclude metastatic disease [40]". Furthermore, a study from one institution had reported chronologic improvement in disease-free survival after surgery alone, with results similar to those for the combined modality studies [41]. A randomized adjuvant study was therefore undertaken at that institution, comparing surgical amputation to surgery with high-dose methotrexate; no difference in disease-free survival between the two groups was shown [42]. The "indictment of the historical control methodology as a failure" continued to be stressed [43]. The controversy surrounding the use of historical controls in osteogenic sarcoma greatly affected Jaffe: "The opprobrium that existed at that particular time was indeed distasteful [44]". This is how Jaffe summed up the situation: "The effect of the report was profound and tended to gain momentum; it was almost a state of hysteria. It was said that what Jaffe had done and wrote about was inaccurate, was not true. It came to a stage that even my own fellows began to have doubts about the situation. I was a *persona non grata* for five or six years. Finally high dose methotrexate was accepted as an established form of treatment in osteogenic sarcoma. I was vindicated [36]". The author asked Jaffe what was his greatest success, what had given him most satisfaction in his professional life? The immediate reply was unexpected: "The fact that I was right from the very beginning and that I did not deviate from the course. I was not overwhelmed by the major criticisms that were directed against me. I had reviewed and re-reviewed the historical controls and the brilliant responses that occurred with high-dose methotrexate. The therapeutic results were no flukes, they occurred [36]".

The historical control controversy was finally put to rest after two prospective randomized studies initiated in the early 1980s and carried out specifically with the view of testing the role of adjuvant chemotherapy in the treatment of osteogenic sarcoma [45, 46]. One study compared the outcomes of patients treated with amputation only with outcomes for patients who also received a five-drug combination including doxorubicin and high dose methotrexate with leucovorin rescue, and with a historical control group [45]. In the other trial, a comparison was made between amputation only, and amputation followed with a six-drug combination also including doxorubicin and high dose methotrexate with leucovorin rescue [46]. In both studies, pre-treatment work-up was identical for both the patients treated with surgery only and patients receiving combination chemotherapy. Both trials revealed a highly significant increase in survival in favor of the chemotherapy treated groups. Indeed, the conclusion was: "From the results of this study the favorable effect of adjuvant chemotherapy on relapse-free survival in patients with osteogenic sarcoma of the extremity appears incontrovertible [46]". Updates have shown that the positive results of these two studies have been maintained [47, 48].

Ironically, the merit of selecting historical controls in specific circumstances, such as those for which they were used in the initial combined modality studies of osteogenic sarcomas had been convincingly debated and justified the very same year the Cortes' and Jaffe's adjuvant studies were published [49].

REFERENCES

[1]   Frei E 3rd. Prospectus for cancer chemotherapy. Cancer 1972; 30:1656-61.
[2]   Arcamone F, Cassinelli G, Fantini G, *et al.* Adriamycin, 14-hydroxydaunomycin, a new antitumor antibiotic from *S. peucetius* var. *caesius.* Biotechnol Bioeng 1969; 11:1101-10.
[3]   Arcamone F-M. Fifty years of chemical research at Farmitalia. Chem Eur J 2009; 15:7774-91.
[4]   Bonadonna G, Monfardini S, De Lena M, Fossati-Bellani F. Clinical evaluation of adriamycin, a new antitumor antibiotic. Br Med J 1969; 3:503-6.

[5]   Bonadonna G, Monfardini S, de Lena M, Fossati-Bellani F, Beretta G. Phase I and preliminary Phase II evaluation of adriamycin (NSC 123127). Cancer Res 1970; 30:2572-82.

[6]   O'Bryan RM, Luce JK, Talley RW, Gottlieb JA, Baker LH, Bonadonna G. Phase II evaluation of adriamycin in human neoplasia. Cancer 1973; 32:1-8.

[7]   Blum RH, Carter SK, Adriamycin. A new anticancer drug with significant clinical activity. Ann Intern Med 1974; 80:249-59.

[8]   Bagley CM Jr, Young CR, Canellos GP, DeVita VT. Treatment of ovarian carcinoma: possibilities for progress. N Engl J Med 1972; 287:856-62.

[9]   Hreshchyshyn MM. A critical review of chemotherapy in the treatment of ovarian carcinoma. Clin Obstet Gynecol 1961; 4:885-900.

[10] Curreri AR, Ansfield FJ, McIver FA, Waisman HA, Heidelberger C. Clinical studies with 5-fluorouracil. Cancer Res 1958; 18:478-84.

[11] Vaitkevicius VK, Brennan MJ, Beckett VL, Kelly JE, Talley RW. Clinical evaluation of cancer chemotherapy with 5-fluorouracil. Cancer 1961; 14:131-52.

[12] Sullivan RD, Miller E, Zurek WZ, Oberfield RA, Ojima Y. Re-evaluation of methotrexate as an anticancer drug. Surg Gynecol Obstet 1967; 125:819-24.

[13] Wilson WL, Bisel HF, Cole D, Rochlin D, Ramirez G, Madden R. Prolonged low-dosage administration of hexamethylmelamine (NC 13875). Cancer 1970; 25:568-70.

[14] Barlow JJ, Piver MS, Chuang JT, Cortes EP, Ohnuma T, Holland JF. Adriamycin and bleomycin, alone and in combination, in gynecologic cancers. Cancer 1973; 32:735-43.

[15] Wiltshaw E, Kroner T. Phase II study of *cis*-dichlorodiammineplatinum (II) (NSC-119875) in advanced adenocarcinoma of the ovary. Cancer Treat Rep 1976; 60:55-60.

[16] Longo DL, Young RC. The natural history and treatment of ovarian cancer. Ann Rev Med 1981; 32:475-90.

[17] Greenspan EM, Fieber M. Combination chemotherapy of advanced ovarian carcinoma with the antimetabolite, methotrexate, and the alkylating agent, thioTEPA. J Mt Sinai Hosp N Y. 1962; 29:48-62.

[18] Young RC, Chabner BA, Hubbard SP, *et al.* Advanced ovarian adenocarcinoma. A prospective clinical trial of melphalan (L-PAM) *versus* combination chemotherapy. N Engl J Med 1978; 299:1261-6.

[19] Ehrlich CE, Einhorn L, Williams SD, Morgan J. Chemotherapy of stage III-IV epithelial ovarian cancer with *cis*-dichlorodiammineplatinum (II), adriamycin and cyclophosphamide: a preliminary report. Cancer Treat Rep 1979; 63:281-8.

[20] Vogl SE, Berenzweig M, Kaplan BH, Moukhtar M, Bulkin W. The CHAD and HAD regimens in advanced ovarian cancer: combination chemotherapy including cyclophosphamide, hexamethylmelamine, adriamycin, and *cis*-dichlorodiammineplatinum (II). Cancer Treat Rep 1979; 63:311-7.

[21] Piver MS, Barlow JJ, Lele SB. Incidence of subclinical metastasis in stage I and II ovarian carcinoma. Obstet Gynecol 1978; 52:100-4.

[22] Griffiths CT. Surgical resection of tumor bulk in the primary treatment of ovarian carcinoma. Natl Cancer Inst Monogr 1975; 42:101-4.

[23] Magrath IT, Lwanga S, Carswell W, Harrison N. Surgical reduction of tumour bulk in management of abdominal Burkitt's lymphoma. Br Med J 1974; 2:308-12.

[24] Shapiro DM, Fugmann RA. A role for chemotherapy as an adjunct to surgery. Cancer Res 1957; 17:1098-1101.

[25]   Hyde L, Wolf J, McCraken S, Yesner R. Natural course of inoperable lung cancer. Chest 1973; 64:309-12.

[26]   Wolf J, Patno ME, Roswit B, D'Esopo N. Controlled study of survival of patients with clinically inoperable lung cancer treated with radiation therapy. Am J Med 1966; 40:360-7.

[27]   Hansen HH. Should initial treatment of small cell carcinoma include systemic chemotherapy and brain irradiation? Cancer Chemother Rep 1973; 4:239-41.

[28]   Jackson DV Jr, Richards F 2nd, Cooper MR, *et al*. Prophylactic cranial irradiation in small cell carcinoma of the lung. A randomized study. JAMA 1977; 237:2730-3.

[29]   Fox W, Scadding JG. Medical Research Council comparative trial of surgery and radiotherapy for primary treatment of small-celled or oat-celled carcinoma of bronchus. Ten year follow-up. Lancet 1973; 2:63-5.

[30]   Broder LE, Cohen MH, Selawry OS. Treatment of bronchogenic carcinoma. II. Small cell. Cancer Treat Rev 1977; 4:219-60.

[31]   Livingston RB. Small cell carcinoma of the lung. Blood 1980; 56:575-84.

[32]   Livingston RB, Moore TN, Heilbrun L, *et al*. Small-cell carcinoma of the lung: combined chemotherapy and radiation. A Southwest Oncology Group Study. Ann Intern Med 1978; 88:194-9.

[33]   Johnson BE, Grayson J, Makuch RW, *et al*. Ten-year survival of patients with small-cell lung cancer treated with combination chemotherapy with or without irradiation. J Clin Oncol 1990; 8:396-401.

[34]   Cortes EP, Holland JF, Wang JJ, Sinks LF. Doxorubicin in disseminated osteogenic sarcoma. JAMA 1972; 221:1132-8.

[35]   Jaffe N, Paed D. Recent advances in the chemotherapy of metastatic osteogenic sarcoma. Cancer 1972; 30:1627-31.

[36]   Author's interview with Dr. Norman Jaffe.

[37]   Jaffe N, Frei E III, Traggis D, Bishop Y. Adjuvant methotrexate and citrovorum- factor treatment of osteogenic sarcoma. N Engl J Med 1974; 291:994-7.

[38]   Cortes EP, Holland JF, Wang JJ, *et al*. Amputation and adriamycin in primary osteosarcoma. N Engl J Med 1974; 291:998-1000.

[39]   Sutow WW, Sullivan MP, Fernbach DJ, Gangir A, George SL. Adjuvant chemotherapy in primary treatment of osteogenic sarcoma. A Southwest Oncology Group Study. Cancer 1975; 36:1598-1602.

[40]   Carter SK. The dilemma of adjuvant chemotherapy for osteogenic sarcoma. Cancer Clin Trials 1980; 3:29-36.

[41]   Taylor WF, Ivins JC, Dahlin DC, Edmonson JH, Pritchard DJ. Trends and variability in survival from osteosarcoma. Mayo Clin Proc 1978; 53:695-700.

[42]   Edmonson JH, Green SJ, Ivins JC, *et al*. A controlled pilot study of high dose methotrexate as postsurgical adjuvant treatment for primary osteosarcoma. J Clin Oncol 1984; 2:152-6.

[43]   Carter SK. Adjuvant chemotherapy in osteogenic sarcoma: the triumph that isn't? J Clin Oncol 1984; 2:147-8.

[44]   Pearson M. Historical perspective of the treatment of osteogenic sarcoma: an interview with Dr Norman Jaffe. J Pediatr Oncol Nurs 1998; 15:90-4.

[45]   Eilber F, Giuliano A, Eckardt J, Patterson K, Moseley S, Goodnight J. Adjuvant chemotherapy for osteogenic sarcoma: a randomized prospective trial. J Clin Oncol 1987; 5:21-6.

[46]   Link MP, Goorin AM, Miser AW, *et al*. The effect of adjuvant chemotherapy on relapse-free survival in patients with osteogenic sarcoma of the extremity. N Engl J Med 1986; 314:1600-6.

[47]   Link MP. The multi-institutional osteogenic sarcoma study: an update. Cancer Treat Res. 1993; 62:261-7.

[48]   Bernthal NM, Federman N, Eilber FR, *et al*. Long-term results (>25 years) of a randomized, prospective clinical trial evaluating chemotherapy in patients with high-grade, operable osteo- sarcoma. Cancer 2012; 118:5888-93.

[49]   Gehan EA, Freireich EJ. Non-randomized controls in cancer clinical trials. N Engl J Med 1974; 290:198-203.

Therapeutic Revolution, 2014, 157-180

"My personal therapeutic journey has witnessed an extraordinary growth in drug treatments for pain and other symptoms. The challenge of educating others on their use remains". Dame Cicely Saunders.

"The formal beginning of psycho-oncology dates to the mid-1970s, when the stigma making the word 'cancer' unspeakable was diminished to the point that the diagnosis could be revealed and the feelings of patients about their illness could be explored for the first time". Dr. Jimmie C. Holland.

CHAPTER 13

From Mathematical Models to Palliative Care and Psycho-Oncology

Pierre R. Band[*]

Department of Medicine, McGill University, Montreal, Canada

Abstract: Several innovations of the 1960s and 1970s influenced the future development of medical oncology. The Goldie-Coldman mathematical model related drug sensitivity to chemotherapy to the spontaneous mutation rate of malignant cells towards drug resistance. It added a new dimension to the scientific evidence for primary systemic therapy of cancer (neoadjuvant), an approach first investigated in osteogenic sarcoma and breast cancer that brought a novel orientation to the treatment of solid tumors. The Norton-Simon mathematical model drew attention to the Gompertzian kinetics of solid tumor growth and to the inference that chemotherapy needed to be intensified after achieving a complete response. The finding that dihydrotestosterone is the active form of testosterone in the prostate and the discovery of the nuclear androgen receptor led investigators to study the basis of progression of prostate cancer to androgen independence; from this research emerged the concept of intermittent androgen suppression for the treatment of prostate cancer. The concept of "total pain", with its physical, emotional, social and spiritual aspects, and the emergence of palliative care and psycho-oncology, opened an entirely new era of cancer care.

Keywords: Goldie-Coldman model, intermittent androgen suppression, Norton-Simon model, total pain, palliative care, psycho-oncology.

***Address correspondence to Pierre R. Band:** Faculty of Medicine, McGill University, Montreal, Quebec H3G 1Y6, Canada; E-mail: pierre.band@gmail.com

THE GOLDIE-COLDMAN MATHEMATICAL MODEL: DRUG RESISTANCE

Two hypotheses have been put forth to explain the possible causes of bacterial resistance to bacteriophages and to antibiotics: 1) Exposure to a bacteriophage or to an antibiotic induces the resistant bacterial variant; 2) The resistant variant arose by spontaneous mutation and pre-existed before exposure. In a classic experiment published in 1943, Luria and Delbrück studied the mechanism of resistance of bacteria to a bacteriophage. These authors provided evidence for the spontaneous mutation theory of resistance, based on theoretical grounds and on an experimental model they developed referred to as the fluctuation test [1]. The same deduction was reached with respect to bacterial resistance to antibiotics [2, 3]: "Resistance is an inherited characteristic, which originates through mutation and whose origin is independent of penicillin treatment [3]". Law, who adapted the fluctuation test to the investigation of resistance of leukemia cells to methotrexate, also concluded: "Mutation and selection constitute the mechanism by which resistant leukaemic cells develop [4]".

In the 1970s, two scientists at the British Columbia Cancer Agency in Vancouver, British Columbia, Doctors James Goldie (Fig. **13.1**), a medical oncologist, and Andrew Coldman (Fig. **13.1**), a mathematician and biostatistician, developed a mathematical model based on the spontaneous mutation theory. They related drug sensitivity to chemotherapy to the spontaneous mutation rate of malignant cells towards drug resistance [5]. The model predicted that resistance to chemotherapy would develop rapidly over a few tumor doublings as a function of the mutation rate and the tumor growth rate, and that combination chemotherapy would effectively reduce the value of the mutation rate to resistance. The authors stressed "the importance of the time factor with respect to the initiation of treatment," and concluded that "chemotherapy should be initiated 'circumstances' permitting, before primary treatment is begun [5]".

Goldie approached Coldman and gave him several papers from the Southern Research Institute. "There was evidence from the experimental work of Skipper and Schabel that the expression of drug resistance tended to be dependent on tumor size. When tumors were small, they did not express drug resistance and could effectively be cured, but as they grew larger, the likelihood that they would be resistant increased, and when they exceeded a critical size, it was virtually certain they would be resistant [6]".

> The link Goldie made was to see how this could be applied in a clinical setting; in particular that the tumor burden related greatly to the likelihood that cures could be achieved by chemotherapy. So by being able to look at all the data, I wrote down a mathematical function about the likelihood that drug resistance would be expressed and related to the size of the tumor, and that this mathematical function was in keeping with the data of Skipper, Schabel and others. Following the publication of our article, DeVita who was at the time Head of the National Cancer Institute invited Goldie and me to make a presentation to his Board of Department Heads. The reception was quite favorable and we were encouraged to explore the issue in more detail. We looked at the joint effects of multidrug and tumor cell loss, and showed that cell loss and differentiation accelerated the process of multidrug resistance. Cell loss and differentiation entails that more cell divisions are required before a tumor achieves a fixed size; each tumor stem cell will have an increased pedigree from the initial tumor progenitor cell. The increased number of divisions implies that the likelihood of a mutation occurring is increased compared to an exponentially growing tumor. It became the tumor age and the process of cell loss and differentiation within the tumor that influenced curability [7].

The Goldie-Coldman model provided a rationale and impetus for a worldwide interest in chemotherapeutic interventions prior to locol-regional treatment of the primary tumor. "Neoadjuvant chemotherapy was not an offshoot of the model; clinical trials of chemotherapy before surgery had already been started. However, the model provided a justification grounded in science that was well understood and recognized. From my perspective it represented an example of the general conclusion you would make, and test in a clinical setting, from the postulate that smaller tumors should be more curable, and that combination chemotherapy should lead to improved cure rates compared to single agents [7]".

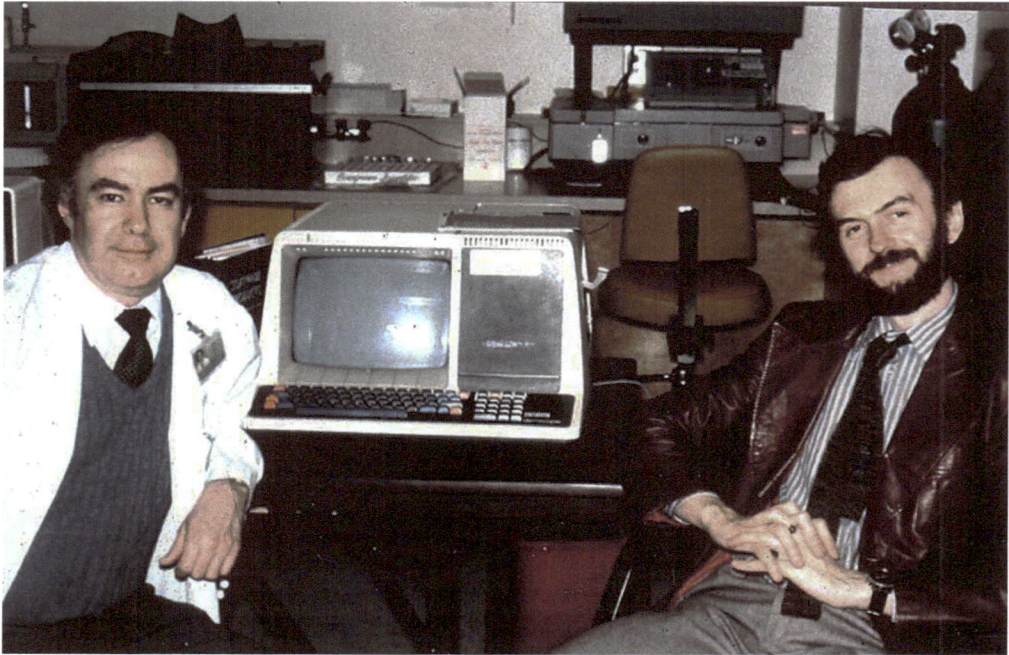

Figure 13.1: Doctors James Goldie (left) and Andrew Coldman, circa 1980. Reproduced with permission from the British Columbia Cancer Research Foundation.

PREOPERATIVE CHEMOTHERAPY

Osteogenic Sarcoma

In the preceding chapter, two postoperative chemotherapy studies following limb amputation were presented: high-dose methotrexate with leucovorin rescue was used in one, doxorubicin in the other. The data prompted Dr. Gerald Rosen (Fig. **13.2**) at the Memorial Sloan-Kettering Cancer Center to combine these drugs preoperatively in an effort to halt tumor growth while a custom internal osseous prosthesis was crafted, thereby preventing amputation. The results were spectacularly successful (James F. Holland, personal communication). Following tumor resection and prosthetic bone replacement, patients also received postoperative chemotherapy [8]. Successive preoperative chemotherapy protocols built on dose-schedule modification and on the addition of new and effective agents led to dramatic improvement in disease-free survival, with 80% of patients with osteogenic sarcoma alive without evidence of disease seven years after initiation of therapy.

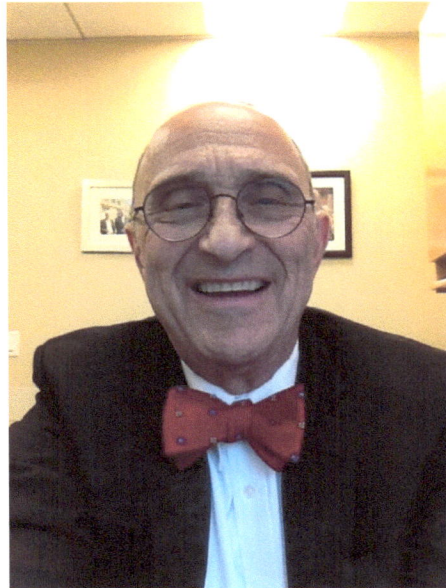

Figure 13.2: Dr. Gerald Rosen. Photo kindly provided to the author by Dr. Rosen.

The primary rationale for preoperative chemotherapy shifted from reducing the size of the primary tumor and awaiting a custom-crafted prosthesis to increasing the cure rate of patients with osteogenic sarcoma [9, 10]. As emphasized by Rosen, neoadjuvant chemotherapy allowed for:

"Definition of drugs and drug combinations that are active in the treatment of a particular disease.

Definition of the dose and timing of administration of those agents that cause optimal regression in the primary tumor and thus are optimal dose schedules to be used in adjuvant chemotherapy after primary tumor surgery.

The early eradication of microscopic foci of metastatic disease and the prevention of resistant clones of tumor cells . . . thus leading to high cure rates [11]".

The osteogenic sarcoma paradigm for neoadjuvant chemotherapy has taught us that the most important prognostic factor for disease-free and overall survival of any disease where neoadjuvant chemotherapy is used is the complete response of the primary tumor (Rosen, personal communication).

Breast Cancer

Chemotherapy prior to radiation therapy of the breast was initiated in 1973 by Bonadonna's group at the National Cancer Institute in Milan, in women with primary inoperable breast cancer [12, 13]. Preoperative chemotherapy of stages I-II breast cancer, however, was pioneered by Dr. Joseph Ragaz (Fig. **13.3**) at the British Columbia Cancer Agency. Ragaz also played a crucial role in spreading the concept internationally.

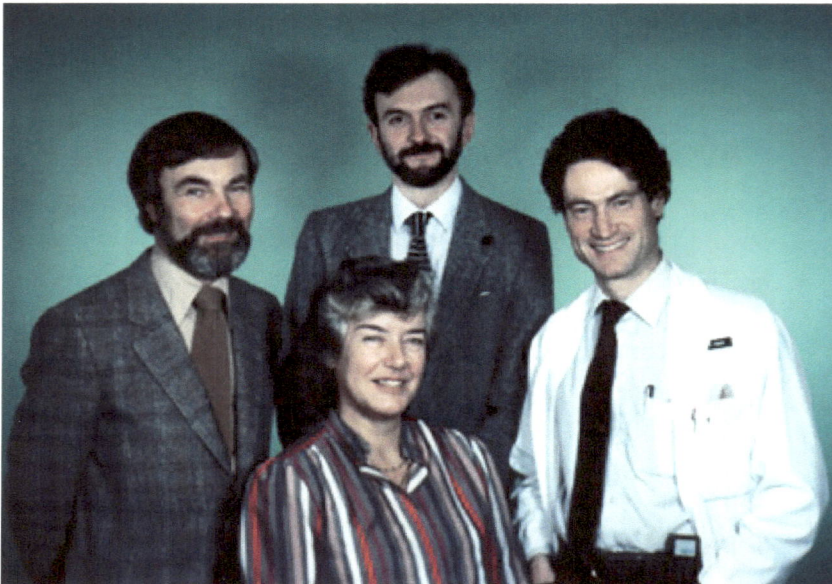

Figure 13.3: From left to right: Doctors Robert Baird, Patricia Rebbeck, Andrew Coldman, Joseph Ragaz. Photograph taken in 1980 kindly provided to the author by Dr. Ragaz with the caption: "The British Columbia Cancer Agency Neoadjuvant Team".

Surgical removal of the primary tumor in the experimental Lewis lung carcinoma model in mice is followed by acceleration of the growth rate of lung metastases [14, 15]. This observation, as well as the beneficial effects reported by the Italian group in advanced breast cancer, motivated Ragaz to use preoperative chemotherapy with a view to abrogating the stimulation of metastatic foci following resection of the primary tumor, and to improving cure rates. The other incentives for preoperative chemotherapy were to assess its downstaging potential, as well as the pathological response to chemotherapy in the mastectomy specimen.

In 1977, Ragaz proposed a pilot project using one cycle of combination chemotherapy prior to surgery for Stages I-II breast cancer. To minimize the possibility of kinetic acceleration of metastases by open surgical diagnostic biopsy, fine needle aspiration was used [16].

The challenges they faced stemmed from the fact that in the late 1970s postoperative adjuvant chemotherapy was not yet a universally accepted policy. At the British Columbia Cancer Agency, after much discussion, postoperative combination chemotherapy was about to be recommended for high risk premenopausal breast cancer patients only. Hence, Ragaz faced opposition in having his preoperative protocol accepted for newly diagnosed cases with early breast cancer. "I was a heretic and almost excommunicated from the Agency [17]". Authorization was finally received for one course of preoperative combination chemotherapy.

Ragaz presented the rationale and early safety results of the pilot study of preoperative chemotherapy for stages I-II breast cancer at several conferences including a National Institutes of Health Consensus Development Conference [17]. He was also instrumental in organizing the first world symposium on preoperative chemotherapy held in Vancouver in March 1985 [18]. The preoperative chemotherapy torch was passed to the NSABP, which initiated a randomized study comparing preoperative to postoperative chemotherapy in 1988. Preliminary results of this study showed that preoperative chemotherapy decreased the size of breast tumors and the incidence of positive nodes. It was therefore suggested that preoperative chemotherapy be considered as first line therapy for breast cancer too large for lumpectomy [19].

A Point of Semantics

Reasons to use chemotherapy prior to surgery and/or radiation therapy evolved over time from a means of reducing a primary tumor mass, to counteracting potential increased growth rates of metastases following surgery and treating micrometastases as early as possible, as suggested by the Goldie-Coldman model. Frei coined the term "neoadjuvant" for this novel therapeutic approach in his David A. Karnofsky Memorial Lecture: "The relatively new concept that I will address involves the use of chemotherapy initially . . . I will refer to this approach as neoadjuvant chemotherapy [20]".

Six years later, Frei provided additional justifications for his choice of the word neoadjuvant that had remained controversial. He considered that: "The term adjuvant chemotherapy has gradually become, and is today universally accepted" and "The novel therapeutic opportunities suggested that the best term should emphasize the novelty of the concept and approach—hence 'new' adjuvant or neoadjuvant [21]".

The author indicated in Chapter 11 that the term adjuvant described a limited and specific situation: the use of a very short course of chemotherapy to destroy cells disseminated in the blood stream during surgery. Under these circumstances adjuvant chemotherapy represented an ancillary, auxiliary or secondary measure to assist surgery. The term was no longer appropriate for studies with a curative intent that aimed to destroy micrometastatic foci left after removal of the primary tumor. The neologism "neoadjuvant" is even more unfortunate as applied to chemotherapy before surgery and/or radiation therapy; in this situation, surgery and/or radiation therapy are in fact adjuvants to chemotherapy. A more appropriate term would be "primary therapy," which not only reflects a principal role in relation to surgery and/or radiation therapy, but is applicable to any form of *systemic* therapy used as an initial modality, for example primary chemotherapy, primary hormonotherapy or primary immunotherapy.

Primary systemic therapy represents a new orientation in the treatment of operable solid tumors. It offers ground-breaking therapeutic possibilities similar in nature to those that led to the cure of childhood acute leukemia. Innovative clinical trials will be generated that will lead to higher proportions of preoperative complete pathology responses, and increased duration of postoperative complete clinical remissions that will no doubt result in major improvement in the survival of patients with solid tumors.

THE NORTON-SIMON MATHEMATICAL MODEL: KINETIC RESISTANCE

In 1977 Doctors Larry Norton (Fig **13.4**) and Richard Simon drew attention to the fact that the exponential model of tumor growth derived from the experimental L1210 leukemia and successfully used for the treatment of childhood acute leukemia did not generally apply to solid tumors. They pointed out in particular that patients with Hodgkin's disease induced into complete remissions with combination chemotherapy may develop recurrences at the initial sites of involvement and retain sensitivity to the same drug combination; clearly biochemical drug resistance could not be a factor in this situation. The authors also commented on the resistance to chemotherapy of large tumors and concluded: "Clinical experience suggests that some tumors may be less sensitive to therapy when they are very small or very large than when they are of intermediate size". Norton and Simon, therefore, developed a model derived from the Gompertz function that described solid tumor growth more accurately than the exponential model [22].

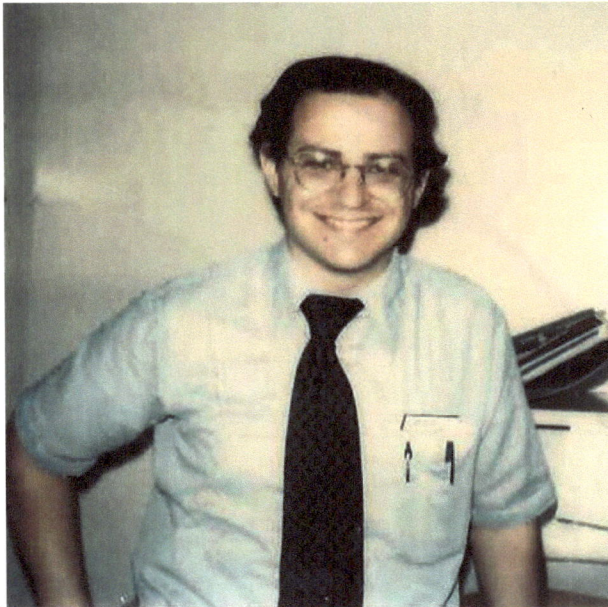

Figure 13.4: Dr. Larry Norton at the time the model was conceived. Photo kindly provided to the author by Dr. Norton.

They noted that for the Gompertzian model "the growth rate is smallest for both very small and very large tumors, and is maximum at a point called the 'inflection point' when the tumor is about 37% of its maximum size" (Fig. **13.5**), and suggested that the effectiveness of chemotherapy is proportional to the growth rate of an untreated tumor at a given tumor size [22].

Since the growth rate decreases as tumor grows above the inflection point and from the inflection point towards smaller tumor volumes, Norton and Simon inferred from their model that chemotherapy should be intensified following induction of a complete tumor response when tumor volumes would presumably be below the inflection point.

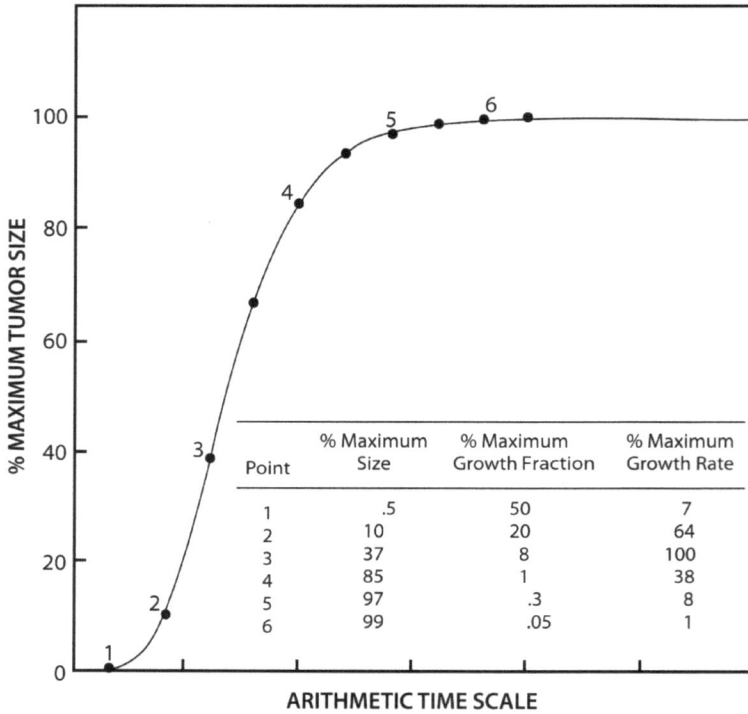

Point	% Maximum Size	% Maximum Growth Fraction	% Maximum Growth Rate
1	.5	50	7
2	10	20	64
3	37	8	100
4	85	1	38
5	97	.3	8
6	99	.05	1

Figure 13.5: (Fig. **2**) in: Norton L, Simon R. Tumor size, sensitivity to therapy, and design of treatment schedules. Cancer Treat Rep 1977; 61; 1307-17, reference 22. Reproduced with permission from NIH INFO.

As shown in Fig 13.5, the percentage maximum growth rates of points 1 and 5 are similar, but their respective percent maximum growth fractions differ widely. In Chapter 5, we referred to the work of Bruce which provided a rationale for drug selection with respect to tumor growth rates [23]. It would seem that in the context of the Norton-Simon model, a combination of predominantly cell-cycle specific drugs should be used against small tumor volumes. For larger tumor volumes, predominantly cell-cycle nonspecific agents should be contemplated or, possibly, cell-cycle specific drugs to eradicate proliferating cells and recruit non-proliferating cells into cycle [24]. Primary chemotherapy would appear to be the optimal setting to clinically assess the therapeutic implications of kinetic resistance suggested by Norton and Simon, with different approaches prior to surgery when tumor volumes are large, and postoperatively when tumor volumes are smaller. It may be anticipated that the therapeutic challenges of drug and kinetic resistance will be simultaneously addressed in future clinical trials.

THE ORIGIN OF INTERMITTENT ANDROGEN SUPPRESSION IN PROSTATE CANCER THERAPY

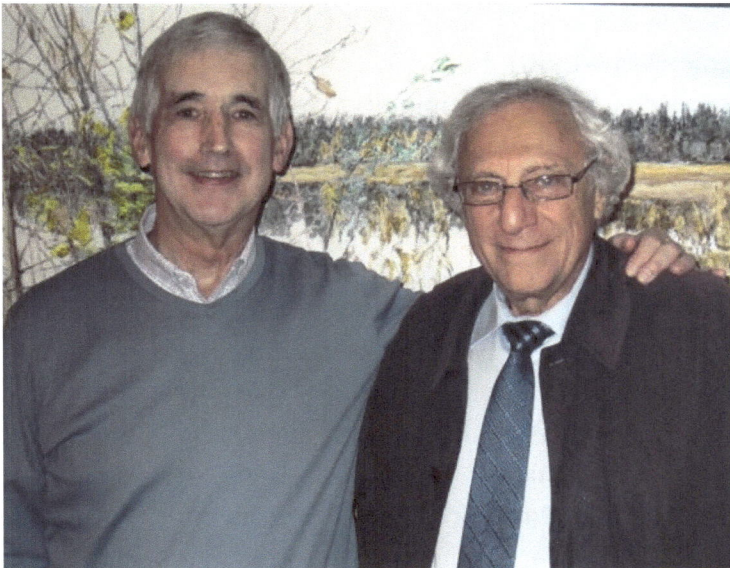

Figure 13.6: Doctors Nicholas Bruchovsky (left) and Pierre R. Band; Vancouver, 2012. Author's collection.

In his final year of medical school at the University of Toronto, Ontario, Nicholas Bruchovsky (Fig. **13.6**) attended a lecture by Dr. Vera Peters (1911-1993), who was well known for her work in Hodgkin's disease and breast cancer [25, 26]. She discussed the effects of hormonal therapy on malignancies and triggered Bruchovsky's interest in the endocrine aspects of oncology. Dr. Bruchovsky later became a resident and fellow with Dr. Jean Wilson in the Endocrinology Division, Department of Internal Medicine, at the Southwestern Medical School in Dallas, Texas. Within a few months, Bruchovsky showed that dihydrotestosterone is the active form of testosterone in the prostate [27, 28] and was the first to describe the nuclear androgen receptor [29].

On his return to Canada, Bruchovsky started a long-term research program at the University of Alberta in Edmonton, which was later continued at the British Columbia Cancer Agency, on the effects of androgens and androgen suppression on the normal prostate gland [30-32]. Two areas were of special interest: the induction of autophagic lysis, later called apoptosis, and the endocrinology of tumor progression [33-35].

"My thinking was influenced by the work of Doctors Leslie Foulds (1902-1974) and Robert Noble (1910-1990); both had emphasized that therapies based on the ablation of hormones, although initially resulting in a dramatic response, increased the rate of progression to autonomous growth [36, 37]. In addition, clinical experience had shown that it was possible to induce multiple regressions of breast cancer in women with a succession of hormonal manipulations [34]. Would it be possible, therefore, to devise a therapy for an endocrine-related cancer that would produce multiple regressions without accelerating progression to autonomy [38]?" It was observed that residual cells in the prostate after castration underwent from one to four divisions during the regrowth of the gland back to its normal size under the influence of dihydrotestosterone, and that in the absence of the hormone to sustain growth, cell death would supervene again [31, 32]. "This implied that more than one round of tissue regression was only possible if androgen-deprived cells were induced to undergo anywhere up to four divisions under the influence of dihydrotestosterone. This seemed to be necessary to rebuild the potential for autophagic lysis of a prostatic cell [38]".

At the same time, Bruchovsky was carrying out experiments with the Shionogi carcinoma, an androgen-dependent mouse mammary carcinoma [39], hoping that it would mimic the clinical behaviour of prostate cancer. In those days, whether a tumor was androgen-dependent was defined largely by its ability to grow in a male animal but not in a female or in a castrated male, whereas from a clinical point of view, an androgen-dependent tumor was one that regressed when androgen was withdrawn. "A hormone-dependent variant obtained from

Dr. William Meakin at the Ontario Cancer Institute was chosen as it required androgens for growth, underwent castration-induced regression, and was characterized by autonomous growth when it recurred [33, 35, 38]". Bruchovsky devised an *in vivo* limiting dilution assay to measure the changes in the fraction of tumorigenic stem cells in the Shionogi carcinoma in response to castration. Castration produced a massive increase in the proportion of androgen-independent stem cells in the previously androgen-dependent malignancy [35]. In a follow-up experiment, the androgen-dependent tumor was transplanted into normal male mice that were castrated six days later. When the tumor regressed to about 30% of its weight, it was removed and transplanted to another non-castrated male mouse. This cycle could be repeated five times over a period of 160 days before progression to androgen-independent growth was observed, whereas without these cycles, tumor autonomy emerged after 50 days [40]:

> The reason that cycles of androgen withdrawal and replacement, that is intermittent androgen suppression, were effective is that the emergence of androgen-independent stem cells was delayed [41]. This added strength to the idea that the same approach might be used to decrease the rate of progression to androgen independence in patients [40]. However, it was not possible to formally test the concept of intermittent androgen suppression in the treatment of prostate cancer in man until the availability in the early 1980s of medical castration with antiandrogens and gonadotropin releasing hormone agonists and of prostate-specific antigen for monitoring the effects [38].

In a Phase II trial of medical castration with antiandrogens initiated in 1983, treatment was interrupted in six patients. Two of them were singers who wished to recover their normal voice temporarily for a concert; none of the six patients experienced any adverse effects [42]. Subsequently, the regimen of repeated cycles of androgen withdrawal and replacement with prostate-specific antigen surveillance was instituted in seven patients. The report on this study [40] attracted worldwide interest and stimulated many clinical trials [43]. Subsequent overviews have reported that intermittent androgen suppression is as effective as continuous androgen suppression therapy in terms of time-to-disease progression and survival, but superior with regard to quality of life and improved sexual function. It was concluded that intermittent androgen suppression should be offered as standard therapy in most patients with nonmetastatic prostate cancer requiring hormonal therapy and in selected cases of metastatic disease [44, 45].

It is interesting to note that in British Columbia, mortality rates from prostate cancer remained fairly stable between 1970 and 1990, ranging from 25.8 per 100,000 to 28.1 per 100,000, suggesting that surgery, radiation therapy, surgical castration, estrogen hormones and prostate-specific antigen (little used at that time) had no impact. Since 1990, prostate cancer mortality rates have declined by one-third, from 28.1 per 100,000 to 18.6 per 100,000, in 2010 (British Columbia data provided to the author by Dr. Andrew Coldman and Norman Phillips). Intermittent androgen suppression, which was initiated in British Columbia in 1986, likely played a role in the downward mortality trend.

The author met Bruchovsky on July 1, 1969 at the entrance to the Clinical Sciences Building at the University of Alberta in Edmonton; by coincidence our two offices were adjacent to each other. Bruchovsky was a prolific writer, but the way he proceeded, was puzzling. His desk was cluttered with very short pencils, each hardly more that a piece of lead attached to an eraser. He would take one at random, write a couple of sentences, then look for another pencil stub to erase certain words and pick-up a different one to write again. The author feels that he made a significant contribution to his friend's career by suggesting that he should use only one full-length pencil to make his writing keep pace with the flow of his thoughts.

PAIN: THE ROOT OF PALLIATIVE CARE

"The physician should use morphine as a miser spends his gold". This instruction appears on page 249 of the second edition (1955) of *The Pharmacological Basis of Therapeutics*, by L.S. Goodman and A. Gilman, the classic pharmacology textbook, currently in its 12th edition. All North American medical students, including the author, were nurtured by that book. This is how generations of physicians viewed morphine, and it is why many cancer patients were left with uncontrolled pain. This situation would slowly change with the vocation of physicians whose focus was to care for the dying.

Dame Cicely Saunders, St Christopher's Hospice, London, England

Dame Cicely Mary Strode Saunders (1918-2005), (Fig. **13.7**), was a nurse and a social worker. She became a physician and founded St Christopher's Hospice, the first modern hospice in the world, where she devoted her life to the care of dying patients. She drew attention to the proper use of oral morphine, stressing that repeated and regular administration, titrated to the patient's needs to control pain, produced neither dependence nor respiratory depression. She developed the concept of "total pain" with its physical, emotional, social and spiritual aspects. [46].

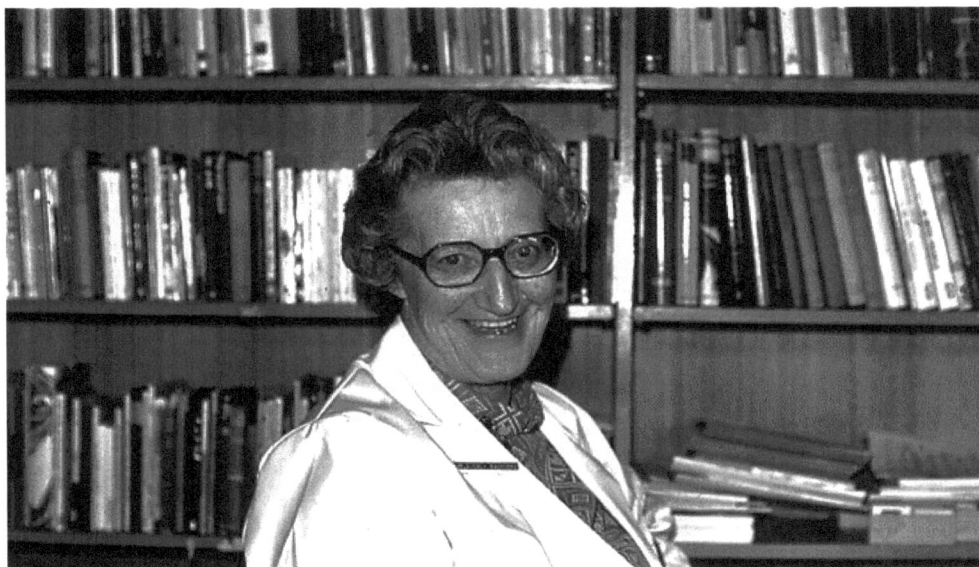

Figure 13.7: Dame Cicely Saunders. Photo kindly provided to the author by Dr. Balfour Mount.

In 1947, while working as a medical social worker, she cared for a Polish Jew, a survivor of the Warsaw ghetto, who died at the age of 40 from a rectal cancer. That crucial encounter marked the beginning of her mission. "During our many talks we discussed somewhere other than that hectic surgical ward that would be more suited to his need for symptom control and the chance to come to terms with his brief and, he thought, useless life. It became a commission for my own future. Leaving me a small legacy he said, 'I'll be a window in your Home' and, on another occasion he said 'I want what is in your mind and in your heart'. When he died, having made his peace with the God of his fathers, I knew he had finished his own journey in the freedom of the spirit [47]".

What Dame Cicely Saunders did not mention was how her own heart and mind helped the patient to end his life in peace. Her influence in the development of palliative care worldwide has been immense. To quote Dr. Balfour Mount: "In terms of palliative care, Cicely Saunders changed the world [48]".

Dr. Balfour Mount, Royal Victoria Hospital, Montreal, Canada

Dr. Balfour Mount (Fig. **13.8**), a urologist, had little notion about death and dying when, in January 1973, he was invited by his local church to chair a panel to discuss the book *On Death and Dying* by Dr. Elisabeth Kübler-Ross (1926-2004). As the evening was being planned, it was suggested that a survey be conducted on how patients died at the Royal Victoria Hospital, the main teaching hospital of McGill University, where Mount was practicing [48]. So a survey of patients, family and staff was carried out to seek their opinion [49]:

> I was shocked by the results. There was poor control of pain and of other symptoms, neglect and isolation and abandonment, desperately inadequate communication with patients and their family; it was not occasionally; it was every case, all the time. It became clear that there was a serious health care problem for patients dying in our hospital that we were largely unaware of and I became interested in seeing what could be done about it. In the book of Kübler-Ross, I noted a number of references with interesting titles from a doctor named Cicely Saunders. Clearly there was someone looking at the needs of the dying; I called Dr. Saunders asking if I could visit her institution. She replied: "I know you; you want to come over with your wife, have a quick run around the house and then go to some plays in London. Well, I won't have it. I tell you what; leave your wife at home, come for a week, plan to roll your sleeves and get involved, and I will have you". I immediately fell in-love with this woman! I visited St Christopher's Hospice; the level of competence of the team and the quality of care was extraordinarily impressive to me. I realized, however, that St Christopher's Hospice was serving a very tiny fraction of the London population and while the care given was phenomenal, it was not in my assessment a cost effective solution to meet the needs of the 80% of patients who, in the Western

World, died in hospitals or home care institutions. So I thought of developing a pilot project to see if a program similar to what Saunders had done could be duplicated in a teaching hospital setting and totally integrated into the health care system. The pilot project was approved and began in January 1975. I wanted to call it hospice, but was told that in French, the word hospice had a connotation with poor medical care. I then thought of palliative and found in the Oxford dictionary that palliative comes from *pallium*, the short cloak that the Romans had to conceal their sword; so *pallium* initially took in Latin the meaning of to hide, to conceal; however, as the word evolved, it turned out to mean to improve the quality of. Now I thought, this exactly defines what Saunders had done, improving the quality of care of the dying. We thus called our program Palliative Care Unit; we modelled it on St Christopher's Hospice, but were the first to apply the lessons learned from Saunders to patients within the setting of a general hospital [48].

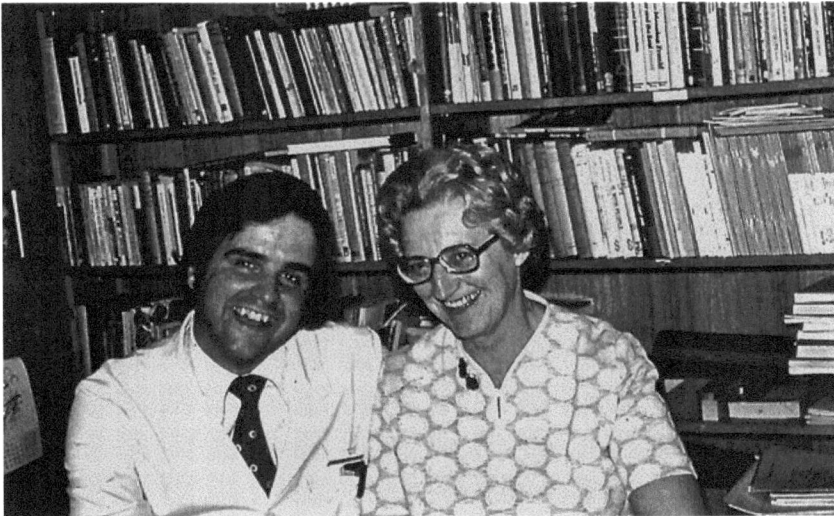

Figure 13.8: Doctors Balfour Mount and Cicely Saunders. Photo kindly provided to the author by Dr. Mount.

A crucial aspect of the scientific approach to pain management was the development of reliable and validated tools, such as the verbal rating scale, the visual analogue scale and the McGill Pain Questionnaire, to objectively evaluate pain and the effect of pain medication [50, 51]. Of these, the visual analogue scale is of special interest. It generally consists of a 0 to 10 cm line with anchor words at each end such as "no pain" and "excruciating pain". The patient marks a point on the line corresponding to the perceived amount of pain. Quantification is made by measuring the distance from the first anchor word ("no pain") to the mark. The visual analogue scale is easy to administer, easy to understand and to score, and is sensitive to variations in pain intensity. Furthermore, it is a ratio scale that expresses pain intensity quantitatively; for example, it makes it possible to conclude that a score of four reflects twice as much pain than a score of two [51]. Of added importance, the realization that subjective symptoms could reliably be measured was paralleled by a growing consciousness and recognition that patients' self reports were dependable and trustworthy.

Sustained-Release Morphine

In 1974, representatives from Napp Pharmaceutical Ltd. and Napp Laboratories in Cambridge, United Kingdom, met with Dr. Robert G. Twycross, who at the time was working with Saunders at St Christopher's Hospice as a Research Fellow in Therapeutics. Napp Laboratories had developed a slow-release system patented as "Continus" which was utilized to develop sustained-release aminophyllin tablets and sustained-release potassium tablets. The firm was considering applying the "Continus" system to a strong opioid as a humanitarian gesture and without any significant commercial expectation; the question posed was which of the strong opioids should be used. Twycross strongly suggested morphine. Napp Laboratories went on to develop "MST Continus", a sustained-release oral preparation of morphine which Twycross evaluated clinically. In the 1980s, MST Continus ultimately accounted for a large proportion of Napp Pharmaceutical sales, which was totally unexpected when the initiative was first conceived (Twycross, personal communication).

Subsequently, Purdue Frederick, Inc. in Toronto, Ontario, made the decision to formally develop the sustained-release product in Canada under the name "MS Contin". John Stewart, who had recently joined Purdue's Clinical Research Group, assumed that responsibility. He approached Mount, who expressed great interest and agreed that the Palliative Care Unit at the Royal Victoria Hospital in Montreal would be a research center for the project [48, 52]. Michèle Deschamps, a research nurse at the Palliative Care Unit, had previous experience in pharmacokinetic studies. She and a pharmacologist from the Université de Montréal, Dr. Jean-Guy Besner, wrote a protocol and initiated a study for the pharmacokinetic assessment of MS Contin. Besner also developed a highly selective, sensitive, and rapid method involving a single step extraction procedure to analyze opiates in human plasma [53].

The pharmacokinetic study did not proceed without concerns and hesitations. Clinical trials had not previously been carried out in the Palliative Care Unit and nothing invasive was done, not even starting an intravenous infusion. So imagine drawing blood every half-hour in terminally ill cancer patients! "The ethics of the situation required careful scrutiny; there were advancements to be gained that required good science. The reason that the study finally got started was because the nursing staff, the patients and their family trusted Michèle Deschamps and the credibility she brought; she was the person who made it happen [48]". After a year Deschamps left the Palliative Care Unit to register as a PhD student; the pharmacokinetic study was subsequently completed with the participation of two other centers using the same protocol [54]. Canadian investigators were the first in North America to perform this type of pharmacokinetic study in cancer patients and obtain approval from the regulatory agency to use MS Contin for the treatment of severe pain requiring the prolonged use of an opioid analgesic [48, 52].

CATASTROPHIC ILLNESS: THE ROOT OF PSYCHO-ONCOLOGY

Dr. Jimmie C. Holland (Fig. **13.9**), a psychiatrist, joined the Memorial Sloan-Kettering Cancer Center in 1977. There, she pioneered the study of psycho-social issues faced by cancer patients and their families and helped them cope with the distress experienced throughout all phases of the disease. She developed programs to help the staff cope with their own distress in caring for cancer patients and established clinical and research training programs in psycho-oncology for nurses, social workers and physicians. She founded and was the first President of the International Psycho-Oncology Society.

> During my internship, I was interested by the way people coped with illness and I went into psychiatry with the idea to study how psychologically

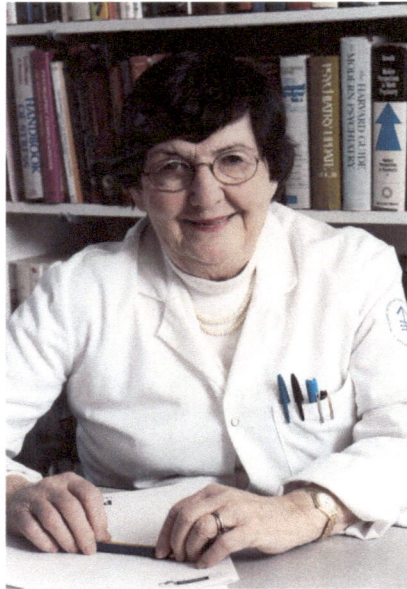

Figure 13.9: Dr. Jimmie C. Holland. Photo kindly provided to the author by Dr. Jimmie C. Holland.

normal people faced catastrophic events. That was fascinating to me. In the course of my training, I was a House Officer at the Massachusetts General Hospital in Boston when the last epidemic of poliomyelitis occurred in the United States. We cleared out a whole ward and replaced hospital beds with iron lung respirators; people were fine one day, paralyzed and unable to breathe the next: an extraordinary catastrophic illness. A colleague and I studied the psychological responses of these patients [55]. Then I married Jim (Dr. James F. Holland), and began to realize that if you want to study how people respond to catastrophic illness, cancer was the disease to study; it affects all ages, all over the world. It was an opportunity to look not only at how individuals cope, but also at the social factors, the beliefs of society that impact on how people cope. The year 1975 was the tipping point: cancer came out of the closet. Some patients were cured of their cancer; there was a wave of optimism; the fear started diminishing; patients became less fearful to say they had cancer. The debate on whether to tell or not to tell patients that they had cancer was beginning. Medicine in general embraced the humanistic side much more and care became more patient centered. So things changed in a positive way in the seventies. This was the time when we began to form a multidisciplinary supportive team for cancer patients and their family; a lot of the early work came out of the efforts of bright nurses who got their PhDs in psychology or other fields [56].

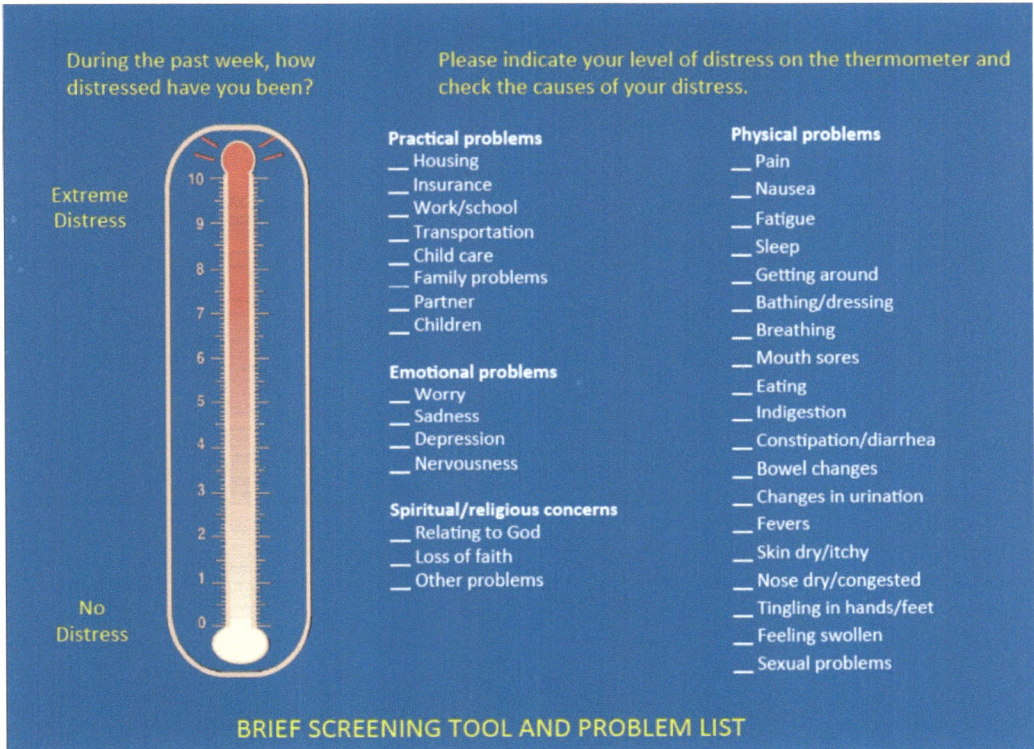

During the past week, how distressed have you been?

Please indicate your level of distress on the thermometer and check the causes of your distress.

Extreme Distress

No Distress

10
9
8
7
6
5
4
3
2
1
0

Practical problems
___ Housing
___ Insurance
___ Work/school
___ Transportation
___ Child care
___ Family problems
___ Partner
___ Children

Emotional problems
___ Worry
___ Sadness
___ Depression
___ Nervousness

Spiritual/religious concerns
___ Relating to God
___ Loss of faith
___ Other problems

Physical problems
___ Pain
___ Nausea
___ Fatigue
___ Sleep
___ Getting around
___ Bathing/dressing
___ Breathing
___ Mouth sores
___ Eating
___ Indigestion
___ Constipation/diarrhea
___ Bowel changes
___ Changes in urination
___ Fevers
___ Skin dry/itchy
___ Nose dry/congested
___ Tingling in hands/feet
___ Feeling swollen
___ Sexual problems

BRIEF SCREENING TOOL AND PROBLEM LIST

Figure 13.10: Distress thermometer scale. Kindly provided to the author by Doctors Jimmie C. Holland and Talia Weiss.

We began the first quality of life studies with the Cancer and Leukemia Group B and it became quite clear that we needed to come up with valid measurements for psycho-social problems; so our first effort was to develop quantitative, validated, reliable patient report scales. We had to prove that patient's self report of their subjective symptoms such as anxiety and depression could be quantified, and scales developed which would allow us to conduct clinical trials of interventions to show their efficacy. A simple approach has been the use of a 0 to 10 scale similar to the visual analogue scale to assess pain; we call this tool the distress thermometer scale (Fig.

13.10); the anchor word "distress" was chosen to reduce the stigma attached to psychological issues. The cut off score for significant distress is 4 or greater. Patients with such scores should be queried further by a member of the oncology team to identify the problem and referred if needed to an appropriate mental health resource. We have done randomized controlled trials using these validated scales and now have evidence bases for several kinds of counselling interventions [57]. In the United States, pain is now officially considered as the fifth vital sign. With the International Psycho-Oncology Society, we recommended that distress should become the sixth vital sign; this recommendation was recently adopted by the International Union against Cancer [56].

Dr. Jimmie C. Holland's efforts culminated in the recognition of psycho-oncology as a distinct specialty of oncology.

REFERENCES

[1]   Luria SE, Delbrück M. Mutations of bacteria from virus sensitivity to virus resistance. Genetics 1943; 28:491-511.
[2]   Newcombe HB. Origin of bacterial variants. Nature 1949; 164:150-1.
[3]   Demerec M. Production of staphylococcus strains resistant to various concentrations of penicillin. Proc Natl Acad Sci USA 1945; 31:16-24.
[4]   Law LW. Origin of the resistance of leukaemic cells to folic acid antagonists. Nature 1952; 169:628-9.
[5]   Goldie JH, ColdmanAJ. A mathematic model for relating the drug sensitivity of tumors to their spontaneous mutation rate. Cancer Treat Rep 1979; 63:1727-33.
[6]   Author's interview with Dr. James Goldie.
[7]   Author's interview with Dr. Andrew Coldman.
[8]   Rosen G, Murphy ML, Huvos AG, Gutierrez M, Marcove RC. Chemotherapy, *en bloc* resection, and prosthetic bone replacement in the treatment of osteogenic sarcoma. Cancer 1976; 37:1-11.
[9]   Rosen G, Marcove RC, Caparros B, Nirenberg A, Kosloff C, Huvos AG. Primary osteogenic sarcoma. *The rationale for preoperative chemotherapy and delayed surgery.* Cancer 1979; 43:2163-77.
[10]   Rosen G, Caparros B, Huvos AG, *et al.* Preoperative chemotherapy for osteogenic sarcoma: *selection of postoperative adjuvant chemotherapy based on the response of the primary tumor to preoperative chemotherapy.* Cancer 1982; 49:1221-30.
[11]   Rosen G. Neoadjuvant chemotherapy for osteogenic sarcoma: a model for the treatment of other highly malignant neoplasms. Recent Results Cancer Res 1986; 103:148-57.
[12]   Zucali R, Uslenghi C, Kenda R, Bonadonna G. Natural history and survival of inoperable breast cancer treated with radiotherapy and radiotherapy followed by radical mastectomy. Cancer 1976; 37:1422-31.

[13]   De Lena M, Zucali R, Viganotti G, Valagussa P, Bonadonna G. Combined chemotherapy -radiotherapy approach in locally advanced (T3b-T4) breast cancer. Cancer Chemother Pharmacol 1978; 1:53-9.

[14]   DeWys WD. Studies correlating the growth rate of a tumor and its metastases and providing evidence for tumor-related systemic growth-retarding factors. Cancer Res 1972; 32:374-9.

[15]   Simpson-Herren L, Sanford AH, Holmquist JP. Effects of surgery on the cell kinetics of residual tumor. Cancer Treat Rep 1976:60:1749-60.

[16]   Ragaz J, Baird R, Rebbeck P, Goldie J, Coldman A, Spinelli J. Neoadjuvant (preoperative) chemotherapy for breast cancer. Cancer 1985; 56:719-24.

[17]   Author's interview with Dr. Joseph Ragaz.

[18]   Preoperative (neoadjuvant) chemotherapy. Ragaz J, Band PR, Goldie JH eds. Recent Results Cancer Res 1985; Vol 103. New York: Springer-Verlag.

[19]   Fisher B, Brown A, Mamounas E, *et al*. Effect of preoperative chemotherapy on local-regional disease in women with operable breast cancer: findings from National Surgical Adjuvant Breast and Bowel Project B-18. J Clin Oncol 1997; 15:2483-93.

[20]   Frei E III. Clinical cancer research: an embattled species. Cancer 1982; 50:1979-92.

[21]   Frei E III. What's in a name-neoadjuvant. J Natl Cancer Inst 1988; 80:1088-9.

[22]   Norton L, Simon R. Tumor size, sensitivity to therapy, and design of treatment schedules. Cancer Treat Rep 1977; 61:1307-17.

[23]   Bruce WR, Meeker BE, Valeriote FA. Comparison of the sensitivity of normal hematopoietic and transplanted lymphoma colony-forming cells to chemotherapeutic agents administered *in vivo*. J Natl Cancer Inst 1966; 37:233-45.

[24]   Valeriote F, van Putten L. Proliferation-dependent cytotoxicity of anticancer agents: a review. Cancer Res 1975; 35:2619-30.

[25]   Cowan DH. Vera Peters and the curability of Hodgkin disease. Curr Oncol 2008; 15:206-10.

[26]   Cowan DH. Vera Peters and the conservative management of early-stage breast cancer. Curr Oncol 2010; 17:50-4.

[27]   Bruchovsky N, Wilson JD. The conversion of testosterone to 5α-androstan-17β-ol-3-one by rat prostate *in vivo* and *in vitro*. J Biol Chem 1968; 243:2012-21.

[28]   Bruchovsky N, Wilson JD. Discovery of the role of dihydrotestosterone in androgen action. Steroids 1999; 64:753-9.

[29]   Bruchovsky N, Wilson JD. The intranuclear binding of testosterone and 5α-androstan-17β–ol-3-one by rat prostate. J Biol Chem 1968; 243:5953-60.

[30]   Bruchovsky N. Comparison of the metabolites formed in rat prostate following the *in vivo* administration of seven natural androgens. Endocrinology 1971; 89:1212-22.

[31]   Lesser B, Bruchovsky N. The effects of testosterone, 5α- dihydrotestosterone and adenosine 3ꞌ , 5ꞌ -monophosphate on cell proliferation and differentiation in rat prostate. Biochim Biophys Acta 1973; 308:426-37.

[32]   Lesser B, Bruchovsky N. The effects of 5α-dihydrotestosterone on the kinetics of cell proliferation in rat prostate. Biochem J 1974; 142:483-9.

[33]   Bruchovsky N, Sutherland DJA, Meakin JW, Minesita T. Androgen receptors: relationship to growth response and to intracellular androgen transport in nine variant lines of the Shionogi mouse mammary carcinoma. Biochim Biophys Acta 1975; 381:61-71.

[34]   Bruchovsky N, Rennie PS, Van Doorn E, Noble RL. Pathological growth of androgen-sensitive tissues resulting from latent actions of steroid hormones. J Toxicol Environ Health 1978; 4:391-408.

[35] Bruchovsky N, Rennie PS, Coldman AJ, Goldenberg SL, To M, Lawson D. Effects of androgen withdrawal on the stem cell composition of the Shionogi carcinoma. Cancer Res 1990; 50:2275-82.

[36] Foulds L. Neoplastic development. New York, Academic Press 1969, volume 1, p. 73.

[37] Noble RL. Hormonal control of growth and progression in tumors of Nb rats and a theory of action. Cancer Res 1977; 37:82-94.

[38] Author's interview with Dr. Nicholas Bruchovsky.

[39] Minesita T, Yamaguchi K. An androgen-dependent tumor derived from a hormone-independent spontaneous tumor of a female mouse. Steroids 1964; 4:815-29.

[40] Akakura K, Bruchovsky N, Goldenberg SL, Rennie PS, Buckley AR, Sullivan LD. Effects of intermittent androgen suppression on androgen-dependent tumors. Apoptosis and serum prostate -specific antigen. Cancer 1993; 71:2782-90.

[41] Akakura K, Bruchovsky N, Rennie PS, Coldman AJ, Goldenberg SL, Tenniswood M, Fox K. Effects of intermittent androgen suppression on the stem cell composition and the expression of the TRPM-2 (clusterin) gene in the Shionogi carcinoma. J Steroid Biochem Mol Biol 1996; 59:501-11.

[42] Goldenberg SL, Bruchovsky N. Use of cyproterone acetate in prostate cancer. Urol Clin North Am 1991; 18:111-22.

[43] Abrahamsson P-A. Potential benefits of intermittent androgen suppression therapy in the treatment of prostate cancer: a systematic review of the literature. Eur Urol 2010; 57:49-59.

[44] Seruga B, Tannock IF. Intermittent androgen blockade should be regarded as standard therapy in prostate cancer. Nat Clin Pract Oncol 2008; 5:574-6.

[45] Klotz L, Toren P. Androgen deprivation therapy in advanced prostate cancer: is intermittent therapy the new standard of care? Curr Oncol 2012; 19 (Suppl 3):13-21.

[46] Saunders C. Into the valley of the shadow of death. A personal therapeutic journey. Br Med J 1996; 313:1599-1601.

[47] Saunders C. Caring for cancer. J R Soc Med 1998; 91:439-41.

[48] Author's interview with Dr. Balfour Mount.

[49] Mount BM, Jones A, Patterson A. Death and dying. Attitudes in a teaching hospital. Urology 1974; 4:741-8.

[50] Melzack R. The McGill Pain Questionnaire: major properties and scoring methods. Pain 1975; 1:277-99.

[51] Deschamps M, Band PR, Coldman AJ. Assessment of adult cancer pain: shortcomings of current methods. Pain 1988; 32:133-9.

[52] Author's interview with John Stewart.

[53] Besner JG, Band C, Rondeau JJ, *et al*. Determination of opiates and other basic drugs by high-performance liquid chromatography with electrochemical detection. J Pharm Biomed Anal 1989; 7:1811- 7.

[54] Thirwell MP, Sloan PA, Maroun JA, *et al*. Pharmacokinetics and clinical efficacy of oral morphine solution and controlled-release morphine tablets in cancer patients. Cancer 1989; 63:2275-83.

[55] Holland JC, Coles MR. Neuropsychiatric aspects of acute poliomyelitis. Am J Psychiatry 1957; 114:54-63.

[56] Author's intreview with Dr. Jimmie C. Holland.

[57] Holland JC, Weiss T. History of Psycho-Oncology. In: Holland JC, Breibart W, Eds. "Psycho-Oncology" 2nd Edition. New York, Oxford University Press, 2010; pp 1-12.

"The evolution of medical oncology has had a major impact on cancer care worldwide". Dr. Byrl J. Kennedy.

CHAPTER 14

October 16, 1973

Pierre R. Band[*]

Department of Medicine, McGill University, Montreal, Canada

Abstract: Before the subspecialty of medical oncology was established, a few internists and endocrinologists had started projects devoted to the treatment of cancer patients; they also played a crucial role in the creation of the American Society of Clinical Oncology. Medical oncology became a subspecialty under the American Board of Internal Medicine (ABIM) through the persistent efforts of Dr. Byrl J. Kennedy whose key contributions to this endeavor are acknowledged by all. A Subspecialty Examination Committee on Medical Oncology was appointed to prepare guidelines for training and accreditation in this field and to prepare questions for the first examination. On October 16, 1973, 351 candidates passed the examination: the first cohort of certified medical oncologists.

Keywords: Medical Oncology, American Board of Internal Medicine, Subspecialty Examination Committee.

INTRODUCTION

Internists and endocrinologists with an interest in the care of cancer patients were the first to pave the long and arduous road leading to the subspecialty of medical oncology. Among them were Doctors Samuel G. Taylor III (1904-1997), Albert H. Owens Jr., and Byrl J. Kennedy (1921-2003), who wrote on the subject and started medical oncology programs in their respective institutions long before the subspecialty was created [1-3]. In 1957, Taylor set up the Committee on Cancer of the American College of Physicians to promote the role of internists in the management of cancer patients. He also founded a Medical Oncology Section at Rush-Presbyterians-St. Lukes' Medical Center in Chicago, the first medical

*Address correspondence to Pierre R. Band: Faculty of Medicine, McGill University, Montreal, Quebec H3G 1Y6, Canada; E-mail: pierre.band@gmail.com

oncology unit within an academic department of medicine at a medical school in the United States (Doctors Jules Harris and Janet Wolter, personal communications). Internists also played a crucial role in the creation of the American Society of Clinical Oncology (ASCO). The Committee of Cancer, ASCO and, above all, Kennedy, with his vision, experience and sustained efforts, were the prime movers of the subspecialty of medical oncology.

AMERICAN SOCIETY OF CLINICAL ONCOLOGY: THE GROUP OF SEVEN

In 1963, Doctors Arnoldus Goudsmit (1909-2005) and Fred J. Ansfield (1910-1996) discussed the idea of a professional organization that would be designed to meet the needs of physicians who were primarily engaged in the care of cancer patients and clinical cancer research. They shared this view with five other colleagues (Fig **14.1**): Harry F. Bisel (1918-1994), Herman Freckman (1912-2009), Robert W. Talley (dates unavailable), William L. Wilson (dates unavailable), Jane C. Wright (1919-2013).

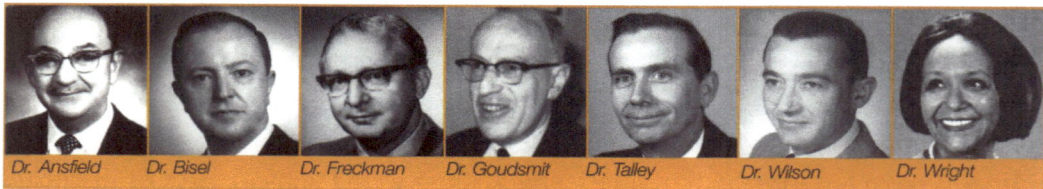

Dr. Ansfield   Dr. Bisel   Dr. Freckman   Dr. Goudsmit   Dr. Talley   Dr. Wilson   Dr. Wright

Figure 14.1: The Group of Seven. ASCO's archival material. Reprinted with permission. © 2011 American Society of Clinical Oncology. All rights reserved.

This group of seven became the Founding Members of ASCO [4-6]. In 1964, the group met to assemble a list of charter members and to draft the constitution and bylaws of the organization. At ASCO's opening meeting on November 5, 1964, attended by 51 physicians, the constitution and bylaws were ratified and Bisel was elected first president of the new society [4-6]. Membership was open to "experienced physicians of any nation who have a predominant interest in the diagnosis and total care of patients with neoplastic disease; and who are directly involved in and responsible for the care of such patients [4]". Kennedy later referred to ASCO as the "voice of medical oncology [7]".

Byrl J. Kennedy

The Masonic Memorial Hospital, now Masonic Memorial Building, dedicated to the care of patients with advanced cancer and to training and research, was inaugurated in October 1958 at the University of Minnesota Medical Center in Minneapolis. In addition to inpatient wards, it included a medical oncology outpatient clinic [8]. Between 1958 and 1966, deploring the "profound lack of adequately trained physicians who are able to act as Medical Oncologists [3]", Dr Byrl J. Kennedy (Fig. **14.2**), B. J. for those who knew him, developed a training program at that hospital for medical students, interns and residents, as well as a specialty training program for physicians wishing to pursue a career in medical oncology. He defined the role of the medical oncologist and the constituents of the medical oncology training program, including epidemiology, tumor biology, detection and diagnosis, patient management, and clinical research [3].

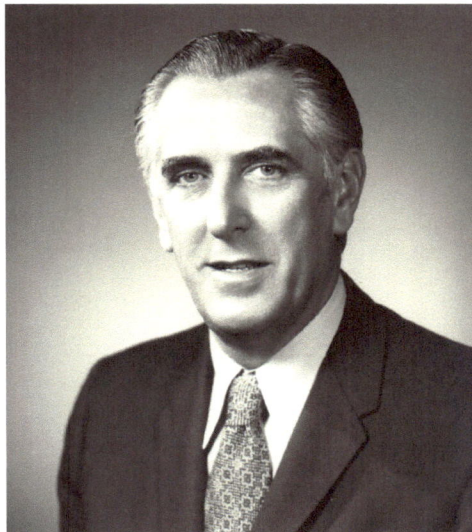

Figure 14.2: Dr. Byrl J. Kennedy; photograph taken in 1973, kindly provided to the author by Dr. Kennedy's children.

On February 20, 1969, Kennedy learned that the American Board of Internal Medicine (ABIM) was modifying training requirements for board certification in internal medicine and subspecialties (Fig. **14.3**). Armed with his experience in

February 20, 1969

Alfred Gelhorn, M. D. , Dean
University of Pennsylvania School of Medicine
Philadelphia, Pennsylvania 19104   Re   Cancer Committee
                                             American College of Physicians
Dear Al:

    I have learned today of the American Board of Internal Medicine's plans to alter the training requirements for the board certification in internal medicine and sub-specialties. As I understand, the future plan would provide for a basic patient-oriented training period of one year as a straight medicine intern and one year as a medical resident. At that time, the fellow can take his basic examinations in internal medicine. Subsequently, he can engage in a minimum of a two or three year program in a sub-specialty. At the end of that period of training, he can take his final examinations which would certify him as a Specialist in Internal Medicine, and at the same time certify him in his chosen subspecialty.

    Currently, cardiology, allergy, and pulmonary diseases are acknowledged sub-specialties. Hematology and probably metabolism will also be seriously considered.

    I believe it would be a major factor for the Cancer Committee of the American College of Physicians, and also the American Society of Clinical Oncology to vigorously promote the acceptance of the subspecialty of Medical Oncology by the American Board of Internal Medicine. In this way, physicians completing training in Internal Medicine and the subspecialty of Medical Oncology will be provided the specialty status that that training program provides. Particularly in view of the hematology status, it is vital that medical oncology maintain an equal circumstance.

    I believe it would be advantageous for us to discuss this as a part of the Cancer Committee Meeting of the American College of Physicians.

    Since I am writing you, may I also just add a slight comment regarding the cancer panel in April. You did this last year, I believe, and I would appreciate your advice on the handling of the mechanics of the cancer panel. This week I will send you a little list of my current ideas on the subject matter and the participants and also ask for your contribution. With best regards,

Cordially,

B. J. Kennedy, M. D.
Professor of Medicine

BJK:kks

Figure 14.3: Letter from Dr. Kennedy to Dr. Gellhorn. ASCO's archival material. Reprinted with permission. © 2011 American Society of Clinical Oncology. All rights reserved.

establishing training programs in medical oncology, his convictions and confidence in his "pioneering, flag-waving program of having the specialty of Medical Oncology recognized throughout the country (Fig. **14.4**)", he stated: "It would be a major factor for the Cancer Committee of the American College of Physicians, and

February 21, 1969

Dr. Sidney Farber
Jimmy Fund Building
Children's Cancer Hospital
Boston, Massachusetts 02115

Dear Dr. Farber:

I am writing regarding my pioneering, flag-waving program of having the specialty of Medical Oncology recognized throughout the country. The American Board of Internal Medicine is altering its specialty requirements so that at the end of a 4 or 5 year training period in internal medicine and subspecialty, that the physician can be certified as a Specialist in Internal Medicine and certified in his chosen subspecialty. Currently pulmonary disease, allergy, and cardiology are already in this category. Hematology and metabolism are also likely candidates.

I would like to promote that Medical Oncology should become a recognized subspecialty in Internal Medicine, warranting certification under the proposed new program. I have written Dr. Alfred Gelhorn in his position as Chairman of the Cancer Committee of the American College of Physicians, and Dr. Emil Frei as President of the American Society of Clinical Oncology.

I would like to have the American Cancer Society consider the merits of recognizing in some way the status of Oncologists, but particularly the subspecialty of Medical Oncology. There certainly also can be the subspecialty of Surgical and Pediatric Oncology. Right now, however, the need to advocate recognition of the Medical Oncology Specialist might be important in providing a larger supply of trained physicians in this area. If the subspecialty does not become certified, I fear that Internal Medicine will lag far behind in accomplishing the attraction of young men into this subspecialty.

I believe the advantage of certification and of adequately trained persons would provide properly qualified specialists for the care of the cancer patient.

I would appreciate your reactions to this proposal. I realize the delicate position that the American Cancer Society is in. I will be at your meeting on March 20th if you would like to discuss it with me at that time.

Cordially yours,

B. J. Kennedy, M. D.
Professor of Medicine
Director-at-Large,
American Cancer Society

BJK:kks

Figure 14.4: Letter from Dr. Kennedy to Dr. Farber. ASCO's archival material. Reprinted with permission. © 2011 American Society of Clinical Oncology. All rights reserved.

also the American Society of Clinical Oncology to vigorously promote the acceptance of the subspecialty of Medical Oncology by the American Board of

Internal Medicine (ABIM) (Fig. **14.3**)". Kennedy's concept was to first define the requirements for an accredited training program in medical oncology to be submitted to ABIM; academic societies implicated in medical oncology were contacted for their support (Fig. **14.5**).

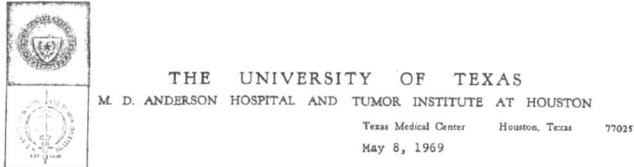

THE   UNIVERSITY   OF   TEXAS
M. D. ANDERSON HOSPITAL AND TUMOR INSTITUTE AT HOUSTON

Texas Medical Center   Houston, Texas   77025
May 8, 1969

Dr. B. J. Kennedy
University Hospital
412 Union Street
Minneapolis, Minnesota 55455

Dear B.J

The Medical Committee on Oncology Subspecialty met in Atlantic City
at 11:00, May 4. Members present included Drs. Gellhorn, Clarkson,
Calabressi, Hall, Steinfeld, Ultmann, and Frei. Initially, we met
with Dr. Brehm, past Chairman of the American Board of Internal Medicine.
Dr. Brehm discussed the recent board changes. These are enclosed.
Dr. Brehm felt that the Board would look favorably upon an application
for formal subspecialty (subsidiary board) in Medical Oncology.

The desirability of having such a subsidiary board was discussed.
It was unanimously agreed that this was desirable. It was proposed
that the training in medical oncology assure enough general training
in internal medicine so that a person completing part I and part II
of training would be in a position to take the general boards in
Internal Medicine as well as the subspecialty boards in Medical Oncology
Drs. Clarkson and Kennedy have already prepared, in writing, material
with respect to the definition of a medical oncologist and his training.
They were requested to prepare joint recommendation along these lines,
and to forward them to Dr. Frei for duplication (through ASCO Resources)
and distribution to members of the committee. All comments will then
be gathered and a final training recommendation will be generated.

It was felt important to get the backing of the various academic
societies involved in medical oncology. The societies and the liason
persons are as follows:

ASCO - Frei; AACR - Holland; American College of Physicians (Cancer
Committee) - Gellhorn; Collaborative Clinical Cancer Therapy Review
Committee - Hall; NCI - Steinfeld; American Cancer Society - Calabressi
and Raul Grant; American Association for Cancer Education - Olson;
and American Cancer Institute Directors - Endicott.

As soon as the training and application proposal is available in
writing, the above persons are requested to consult with appropriate
persons in the above organization to obtain backing.

When the final training recommendation has been reviewed and approved
by the Committee and approval and support obtained from the above
organizations, formal application to the American Board of Internal
Medicine will be made.

Sincerely yours,

Emil Frei, III, M.D.
Associate Director (Clinical Research)

EF:fph

Figure 14.5: Letter from Dr. Frei to Dr. Kennedy. ASCO's archival material. Reprinted with permission. © 2011 American Society of Clinical Oncology. All rights reserved.

Kennedy's leadership in the establishment of medical oncology as a subspecialty of internal medicine is acknowledged by all:

"He carried the torch [9]".

"He led the charge [10]".

"Through hard work and unbending perseverance he and several colleagues . . . convinced the American Board of Internal Medicine (ABIM) to grant medical oncology subspecialty status in 1972 . . . B. J. we owe you much [11]".

"Through the persistent campaigning of Kennedy and his colleagues, medical oncology was established as a subspecialty under the American Board of Internal Medicine (ABIM) [12]".

THE AMERICAN BOARD OF INTERNAL MEDICINE (ABIM) AND THE FIRST EXAMINATION IN MEDICAL ONCOLOGY

Since the 1940s four subspecialties of internal medicine had been certified by ABIM [13]. With subsequent advances in medicine, several requests were submitted for other fields of subcertifications. A Committee on Advanced Examinations was established in October 1969 to oversee the certification of new medical specialties. In December 1970, the committee recommended to the Board that a committee of six members be set up in preparation for an examination in medical oncology. Approval from ABIM and the American Board of Medical Specialties was obtained in February 1971 and February 1972 respectively. A test committee in medical oncology, later called the Subspecialty Examination Committee on Medical Oncology, was approved by the Board in February 1971. The Subspecialty Examination Committee on Medical Oncology was appointed by the Nominating Committee of ABIM to prepare guidelines for training and accreditation in medical oncology and questions for the first examination [13]. The members of this Subspecialty Examination Committee were Doctors Bryl J. Kennedy (Chairman), Paul Calabresi (1930-2005), Paul P. Carbone (1931-2002), Emil Frei III (1924-2013), James F. Holland, and Albert H. Owens Jr. (Fig. **14.6**). The committee defined training requirements in internal medicine and medical oncology required by the candidates and specific to the subspecialty of medical oncology as distinct from the subspecialty of hematology [14]. "Part of the stipulation was that medical oncology was not a subset of hematology, but a discipline in and of itself separate from hematology. Leukemia, for instance, was considered as a cancer of a specific organ not just as a hematologic disease [9]".

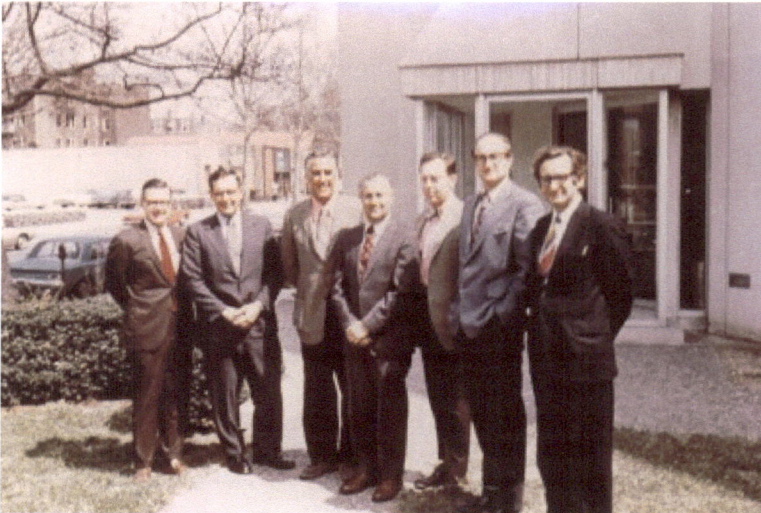

Figure 14.6: The Subspecialty Examination Committee on Medical Oncology. From left to right: Secretary, American Board of Internal Medicine (ABIM), name unavailable; Doctors Paul P. Carbone, Byrl J. Kennedy, Paul Calabresi, Albert H. Owens Jr., Emil Frei III and James F. Holland. Photograph taken outside the ABIM building headquarters in Philadelphia, 1972; kindly provided to the author by Dr. James F. Holland.

The Subspecialty Examination Committee defined general requirements for accreditation in medical oncology and subjects of direct relevance to training in this field, including etiology, tumor biology, epidemiology, detection and diagnosis, patient management, host effects, investigation orientation (clinical trials) and gerontology. These subjects, as indicated above, had been delineated by Kennedy several years before [3]. The members of the committee emphasized that the "chief special skill to be developed is judgment in matters relating to neoplastic diseases [14]". They also came up with questions for the first examination.

"We criticized each other vehemently and finally came out with a decent exam [9]".

"The first Board exam' was a very creative effort; we were not revising anything that had gone on before". (Albert H. Owens Jr., personal communication).

On October 16, 1973, the first examination in Medical Oncology, the ninth subspecialty accredited by ABIM was taken by 478 candidates, of whom 351 (73%) passed [4, 6]: they were the first certified cohort of medical oncologists.

OTHER NATIONS RECOGNIZING THE NEED FOR MEDICAL ONCOLOGY FOLLOWED SUIT.

ANOTHER LANDMARK IN 1973 WAS THE PUBLICATION OF THE FIRST COMPREHENSIVE TEXTBOOK OF MODERN MEDICAL ONCOLOGY (Fig. 14.7).

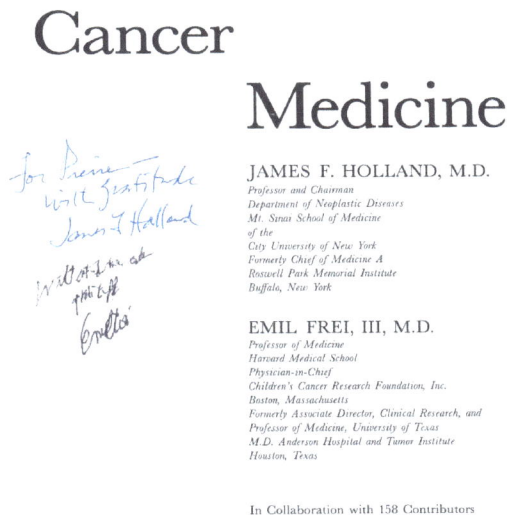

Cancer

Medicine

JAMES F. HOLLAND, M.D.
Professor and Chairman
Department of Neoplastic Diseases
Mt. Sinai School of Medicine
of the
City University of New York
Formerly Chief of Medicine A
Roswell Park Memorial Institute
Buffalo, New York

EMIL FREI, III, M.D.
Professor of Medicine
Harvard Medical School
Physician-in-Chief
Children's Cancer Research Foundation, Inc.
Boston, Massachusetts
Formerly Associate Director, Clinical Research, and
Professor of Medicine, University of Texas
M.D. Anderson Hospital and Tumor Institute
Houston, Texas

In Collaboration with 158 Contributors

LEA & FEBIGER · 1973 · PHILADELPHIA

Figure 14.7: The first edition of "CANCER MEDICINE" autographed in 2010 by Doctors James F. Holland and Emil Frei III. Dr. Frei was severely afflicted with Parkinson's disease at that time. Author's collection.

AN UNEASY ACCOMODATION

The specialty of medical oncology in the United States met with vigorous opposition from most hematologists: "Hematologists were dead set against it [9]". ABIM's approval of a test committee in medical oncology in February 1971 immediately led to discussions with the Board on training for physicians who wanted certification in both medical oncology and hematology. A suggestion was reportedly made by the American Society of Hematology that a single examination be established for both subjects, which the Board did not accept. However, although ABIM continued to support separate certifications, it also eventually approved training for dual certification [13]. The reasons for the acceptance are somewhat clouded:

"Because of overlap with haematology, 3-year training was negotiated for dual certification [15]".

"In May 1974 ASCO revised its position statement to allow for three-year dual certification in special circumstances [6]".

"The Subspecialty Committee on Medical Oncology . . . surprisingly . . . included an unlikely compromise . . . they now grudgingly acknowledged that a 3-year program that included adequate training in medical oncology was a viable alternative. The ABIM revised its training requirements to include dual certification in hematology and oncology [12]".

Despite the opposition and the unclear reasons for the acceptance of dual certification, medical oncology prevailed in the United States.

REFERENCES

[1]   Taylor SG 3rd, Slaughter D. The physician and the cancer patient. JAMA 1952; 150:1012-15.
[2]   Owens AH. A training and research program in medical oncology. Postgrad Med 1961; 29:522-4.
[3]   Kennedy BJ. Training in medical oncology. Arch Intern Med 1968; 121:189-91.
[4]   History of ASCO Monograph. Am Soc Clin Oncol 2004; pp 6-10.

[5]   Krueger GM, Alexander LL, Whippen DA, Balch CM. Arnoldus Goudsmit, MD, PhD: chemotherapist, visionary, founder of the American Society of Clinical Oncology, 1909-2005. J Clin Oncol 2006; 24:4033-6.

[6]   Krueger GM. The formation of the American Society of Clinical Oncology and the development of a medical specialty, 1964-1973. Perspect Biol Med 2004; 47:537-51.

[7]   Kennedy BJ. Medical Oncology. Its origin, evolution, current status, and future. Cancer 1999; 85:1-8.

[8]   Kennedy BJ, Westerman J. Parahospital, Hospitals. J A Hosp Assoc 1962; 36:38-44 and 56-64.

[9]   Author's interview with Dr. James F. Holland.

[10]   Author's interview with Dr. Emil J. Freireich.

[11]   Muss HB. Byrl James Kennedy, MD. J Clin Oncol 2005; 23:3297-8.

[12]   Krueger G, Canellos G. Where does hematology end and oncology begin? Questions of professional boundaries and medical authority. J Clin Oncol 2006; 24:2583-8.

[13]   American Board of Internal Medicine. Internal Monograph. Kindly provided to the author by Dr Eric S. Holmboe, Chief Medical Officer and Senior Vice President, American Board of Internal Medicine.

[14]   Kennedy BJ, Calabresi P, Carbone PP, *et al.* Training program in medical oncology. Ann Intern Med 1973; 78:127-30.

[15]   Kennedy BJ. Origin and evolution of medical oncology. Lancet 2000; 354:siv41.

"There will come a time when physicians will tell their patients: "Don't worry, it's nothing, it's only a cancer". Conversation with Dr. Lucien Israël.

EPILOGUE

Medical Oncology: An Extraordinary Odyssey

The road travelled from 1948, the year of Sidney Farber's report on remissions of childhood acute leukemia, to October 16, 1973, the date of the first subspecialty examination in medical oncology, was spectacular. Over a short time and with only a few drugs, principles of chemotherapy were developed, cooperative oncology groups were created, the phases of clinical trials were established, innovative therapies and imaginative study designs were conceived, leading to cures in such lethal diseases as pediatric cancers, choriocarcinoma, Hodgkin's disease and testicular cancers, as well as increased survival in a number of hematologic malignancies and solid tumors.

In particular, the prognosis of cancer in children and adolescents has improved remarkably since the advent of chemotherapy and with the progress of therapy that resulted from clinical trials [1-3]. The reduction in mortality rates and the numbers of expected deaths from cancer [4, 5] have been associated with substantial increases in five-year and 10-year survival rates that have been well documented in the United States and other countries [1, 2, 6-10]. By the mid 1990s the 10-year survival rate for all cancers in children and adolescents was 71.8% [7] which must stand as one of the greatest achievements of 20th century medicine.

Depending on such factors as the average growth rate of tumors, the effects of treatment and the fact that pediatric cancers, which are rare, are essentially all cared for in academic institutions, while adult cancers, which are common, are predominantly treated in community settings, it may take years before therapeutic standards arising from clinical trials are disseminated and reflected by decreased mortality rates in the population. For instance, highly effective treatments in rapidly growing tumors as exemplified by childhood acute leukemia, may gain more rapid recognition than would more modest therapeutic gains in slower-growing adult solid tumors. It is informative to look at trends in age-specific mortality rates in the United

States population, as shown in Table **1**, which reveal a marked decline in age groups under 45 and an increase in age groups over 55 [4]. Of particular interest, the decline in cancer mortality rates in the 35-to-44 age group only became evident in 1980, and began to be noticeable later in the age group 45-to-54 age group. The shift to the right of these trends suggests that cancer mortality rates will continue to decline overall and among older age groups as therapeutic advances, earlier diagnosis, cancer screening and cancer prevention will become more prevalent. Immunotherapy has become an effective treatment modality against cancer and the genetic revolution has entered the field of medical oncology. In the author's opinion, therapeutic breakthroughs resulting from these extraordinary developments will doubtless be reflected in increased cancer cure rates, increased survival from cancer, and declining cancer mortality rates in all age groups.

Table 1: Cancer mortality rates, 1970 to 1984, United States. Modified from Table **1** in: Breslow L, Cumberland WG. Progress and objectives in cancer control. JAMA 1988; 259: 1690-4, reference 4.

Age Groups	Percent of 1960 Rates		
	1970	**1980**	**1984**
All, age adjusted	3.3	5.6	6.1
<1	-34.7	-55.6	-56.9
1-4	-31.2	-58.7	-63.3
5-14	-11.8	-36.8	-47.1
15-24	0.0	-24.1	-33.7
25-34	-15.4	-29.7	-33.3
35-44	0.3	-18.6	-21.9
45-54	3.1	1.7	-3.7
55-64	6.6	9.9	13.0
65-74	5.7	14.6	17.0
75-84	3.6	9.3	12.9

If past experience predicts the future, we can anticipate that the treatment of premalignant lesions will become one of the most promising branches of medical oncology. That prediction is inescapable from a historical perspective. Indeed, it is revealing to note that progress is moving in parallel with earlier therapeutic interventions. In the beginning, treatment was given to patients with advanced disease, some of whom were moribund with disseminated metastases. New concepts led to postoperative and then to preoperative systemic chemotherapy. With improvements in diagnostic imaging and cancer screening, it became possible to identify and treat more cancers at a curable stage. The next step will be the treatment of premalignant lesions with medicinal agents in order to arrest their progression to overt cancer or to induce their reversal to a more normal pattern, thus reducing the incidence of the major adult solid tumors.

Whatever the future may bring, we must never lose sight of what it was like in the beginning. Reminiscences on the occasion of James F. Holland 65th birthday said it all.

"As in all beginnings, cancer chemotherapy was started by just a few talented and dedicated people with the imagination and audacity to believe that they might succeed in curing human cancer, in the face of many early failures and sometimes not a little derision from their less imaginative colleagues [11]".

"Courage was a necessity in the early days particularly, when everybody was absolutely certain that an investment in the chemotherapy of cancer, and specifically of leukemia, was poor judgement from the research point of view. They were absolutely sure, and 'proved' in a variety of ways, that there was no way to cure cancer. Cynicism masquerading as intelligence was everywhere [12]".

The story of medical oncology was written by men and women of courage, integrity, and conviction, whose ideals, creativity, scientific vision and, above all, passion, led us to where we are today.

REFERENCES

[1]   Hammond GD. The cure of childhood cancers. Cancer 1986; 58 (2 Suppl):407-13.
[2]   Lukens JN. Progress resulting from clinical trials. Solid tumors in childhood cancer. Cancer 1994; 74 (9 Suppl):2710-8.
[3]   Murphy SB. The national impact of clinical cooperative group trials for pediatric cancer. Med Pediatr Oncol 1995; 24:279-80.
[4]   Breslow L, Cumberland WG. Progress and objectives in cancer control. JAMA 1988; 259:1690-4.
[5]   Miller RW, McKay FW. Decline in US childhood cancer mortality. 1950 through 1980. JAMA 1984; 251:1567-70.
[6]   Grovas A, Fremgen A, Rauck A, *et al.* The National Cancer Data Base report on patterns of childhood cancers in the United States. Cancer 1997; 80:2321-32.

[7]   Linabery AM, Ross JA. Childhood and adolescent cancer survival in the US by race and ethnicity for the diagnostic period 1975-1999. Cancer 2008; 113:2575-96.

[8]   Gatta G, Capocaccia R, Coleman MP, Ries LA, Berrino F. Childhood cancer survival in Europe and the United States. Cancer 2002; 95:1767-72.

[9]   Adami H-O, Glimelius B, Sparén P, Holmberg L, Krusemo UB, Pontén J. Trends in childhood and adolescent cancer survival in Sweden 1960 through 1984. Acta Oncol 1992; 31:1-10.

[10]   Ellison LF, De P, Mery LS, Grundy PE. Canadian cancer statistics at a glance: cancer in children. CMAJ 2009; 180:422-4.

[11]   Clarkson BD. Reminiscences. Mt Sinai J Med 1992; 59:377.

[12]   Frei E III. Reminiscences. Mt Sinai J Med 1992; 59:379.

Name Index

A

Alexander S., 26
Ansfield F., 182
Aselli G., 17
Avicenna, 16
Axelrod J., 30

B

Band P., 11, 120, 126,127, 146, 167
Bartholin T., 17
Beatson G., 18, 20, 21
Becquerel H., 18
Beer C., 72
Bertagnolli M., 67
Besner J-G., 175
Bichat M., 17
Bisel H., 182
Bonadonna G., 141, 146, 147, 162
Bruce R., 48, 49, 59, 60, 166
Bruchovsky N., 10, 11, 167-170
Bunche R., 27
Burchenal J., 32, 35, 36, 40, 44, 46, 47, 60, 66, 68
Burkitt D., 100-102

C

Calabresi P., 187, 188
Carbone P., 125, 127, 137, 138, 141, 187, 188
Carter S., 94, 130
Celsus A., 15
Chahinian P., 114
Clarkson B., 65
Coldman A., 10, 158, 160, 162, 170

Z

Subject Index

A

B

www.ingramcontent.com/pod-product-compliance
Lightning Source LLC
Chambersburg PA
CBHW050839220326
41598CB00006B/404